The AHIMA Press *Revenu[e]*
Practices, Second Edition

- Student Ancillaries
- Practice Briefs and Toolkits

How to Register on the <u>Student</u> Website
http://www.ahimapress.org/davis5269/

Scratch off the sticker below to reveal your unique
student code to access the book website. Your access
code and account information cannot be shared or
transferred. Access to the website is for individuals only
and will be terminated on publication of the next edition
of this book.

For access to additional resources, **instructors should
use a unique instructor code,** which will grant access
to both student and instructor resources, rather than
entering the code below.

<u>This book cannot be returned once the code has been
revealed.</u>

Scratch off the sticker with care.

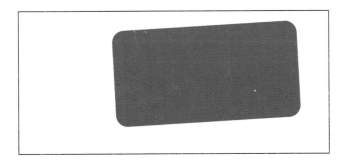

Revenue Cycle Management
Best Practices

Second Edition

Nadinia A. Davis, MBA, RHIA, CHDA, CCS, FAHIMA

and

Belinda M. Doyle, MSJ

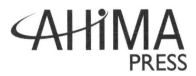

AHIMA PRESS

ISBN: 978-1-58426-526-9

AHIMA Product No.: AB106114

All information contained within this book, including websites and regulatory information, was current and valid as of the date of publication. However, web page addresses and the information on them may change or disappear at any time and for any number of reasons. The user is encouraged to perform his or her own general web searches to locate any site addresses listed here that are no longer valid.

All products mentioned in this book are either trademarks of the companies referenced in this book, registered trademarks of the companies referenced in this book, or neither.

American Health Information Management Association
233 North Michigan Avenue, 21st Floor
Chicago, Illinois 60601-5809
ahima.org

Contents

About the Authors

Nadinia A. Davis, MBA, RHIA, CHDA, CCS, FAHIMA, is the program coordinator of the Health Information Management (HIM) program at Delaware Technical Community College. She was previously an assistant professor of HIM at the College of Natural, Applied, and Health Sciences at Kean University in Union, NJ, and an adjunct instructor of healthcare finance systems in the Health Informatics department at the University of Medicine and Dentistry of New Jersey. She has worked as a coding consultant and auditor in acute settings and as director of medical records at a rehabilitation institute. Her most recent hospital position was as the executive director of revenue cycle for Merit Mountainside Hospital in Montclair, NJ. Prior to her HIM career, Davis worked in the financial services industry, most recently as an internal auditor, and held an active New Jersey certified public accountant license for 20 years, until 2013. She is a former president of the New Jersey Health Information Management Association (NJHIMA) and Delaware Health Information Association (DHIMA), a distinguished member of NJHIMA, and a former member of the American Health Information Management Association (AHIMA) Board of Directors. She is a contributor to *Effective Management of Coding Services* and *Health Information Management: Concepts, Principles, and Practice,* as well as an editor of and contributor to the AHIMA workbook that accompanied Jones & Bartlett's *Essentials of Health Care Finance,* Fourth Edition. She is also coauthor of Elsevier's *Foundations of Health Information Management,* currently in its fourth edition, for which she received an AHIMA Legacy Award.

Belinda M. Doyle, MSJ, is the director of payer services, which includes oversight of the insurance verification and authorization staff, for the 14 locations throughout New Jersey of Children's Specialized Hospital, an affiliate of RWJ Barnabas Health. For 19 years, she has been a professional with diverse financial operations and revenue cycle experience in the healthcare industry, including full-time and consulting roles for hospitals; ancillaries; behavioral health entities; skilled nursing facilities; inpatient acute rehabilitation; pediatric special care nursing facilities (also referred to as long-term care); and professional practices, including dentistry. Her specialty is provider and payer collaboration, which touches every aspect of the revenue cycle, especially the newer pay-for-performance, value-based concepts of reimbursement. Drawing on her keen understanding of the interdepartmental impact of clinical and nonclinical teams on the revenue cycle, she excels at oversight of financial operation committees by specific service line and also oversees denial teams for hospitals and providers. Belinda earned her master's of jurisprudence with an emphasis in healthcare law from Seton Hall Law School. This unique master's degree has afforded her great success in working with payers to ensure that contracts protect the financial operational interests of providers. Her volunteer involvement includes leadership roles in the Healthcare Financial Management Association's New Jersey chapter, such as chairing the payer and provider collaboration committee for two years before being elected to a board of directors position in June 2015, and acting as the board liaison for the Patient Access Services Committee.

Acknowledgments

Many thanks to our families for their support during this project. We thank the reviewers for their valuable insight and suggestions. Thanks to our colleagues—Celia Bosco, esquire, of Genova and Burns Law Firm; Hal E. Clark, partner, River City Health Solutions; Joseph J. Dobosh, Jr., vice president of finance and chief financial officer of Children's Specialized Hospital, an affiliate of RWJ Barnabas Health; Brian Herdman, operations manager, Financial Reimbursement Services of CBIZ K&A Consulting; Gregg Leff, executive vice president of Aergo Solutions; Colleen C. Picklo, project manager and policy analyst of Managed Care of New Jersey Hospital Association (NJHA); and Roger D. Sarao, MPA, CHFP, vice president economic and financial information of NJHA—who answered our questions, read our early drafts, agreed to share materials for our critical thinking exercises, and cheered us on. Everyone's careful reading of the manuscript and thoughtful comments made this a better book than it otherwise would have been. A very special thanks to Nadinia Davis from Belinda for inviting me to be a part of this second edition. It has been fun, and I cannot wait to see what the healthcare industry brings next for the third edition updates.

We also would like to thank in advance the readers of this text. We hope it serves you well.

—**Nadinia A. Davis and Belinda M. Doyle**

Introduction

The purpose of this book is to help health information professionals better understand and participate in revenue cycle management in their facilities. The book focuses primarily on acute-care (short-stay) hospitals and assumes the health information management (HIM) professional view from the perspective of the HIM department. While the authors acknowledge and respect that HIM professionals participate in facility management and operations in myriad roles, the HIM department is the most likely venue from which HIM professionals (absent other training and credentials) will participate in the revenue cycle.

Although an understanding of healthcare financial management is a required competency in the current Commission on Accreditation of Health Informatics and Information Management Education (CAHIIM) baccalaureate curriculum, a focus on accounting and finance beyond budgeting and basic productivity analysis has not always been present in the HIM profession. In an increasingly complex healthcare environment and with many healthcare facilities closing because they are unable to survive bankruptcy, it is important that all healthcare workers understand, appreciate, and participate fully in their role in the financial health of a facility. Since the HIM department directly affects facility reimbursement through the coding function, that function is the most obvious role of the HIM professional in the revenue cycle. However, coding is by no means the HIM professional's only role—hence this book was developed. The authors contend that the days of the "medical record department" being a relatively self-contained silo of activities that pertained solely to postdischarge processing of records ended in 1929, when such departments took on documentation-improvement responsibilities. From that point on, "it's not my (our) job" has not been an acceptable response from HIM professionals to the increasingly complex challenges of the hospital environment.

With respect to this text, the authors do not assume any knowledge of accounting or finance on the part of the reader. Every accounting and financing term is defined and explained, and there is a short accounting primer in chapter 2 that focuses solely on the relationship of the revenue cycle to financial statements.

The authors do, however, assume that the reader has a comprehensive knowledge of healthcare, including clinical services and hospital organizational structure. Pertinent illustrations of specific healthcare issues are included in the text, but explanations of healthcare-related topics are limited to those relevant to the discussion at hand. Further, the authors assume a basic knowledge of reimbursement systems and how they relate to coding. For the benefit of the occasional non-HIM reader, elementary explanations are included and additional resources are listed where appropriate. Bolded terms are defined in the glossary (appendix A).

Anecdotally, it seems that healthcare organizations, particularly those that are not-for-profit, are reluctant to discuss the financial aspects of healthcare delivery with employees. While everyone experiences those financial aspects in their personal lives, the organizational reliance on individuals with minimal financial training and experience to identify, monitor, and complete complicated financial transactions can be crippling. There is a bank that advertises to customers a service in which every transaction posted can be rounded up to a whole dollar amount and the difference placed in savings. The exact opposite is happening in many healthcare organizations. Errors and omissions occur every day and can eventually add up to large, unrecoverable losses for the organization. This is not malicious activity, but rather the result of a lack of understanding. It is the authors' position that every employee needs to understand the revenue cycle of the organization in which he or she works in order to be a truly conscientious, efficient, and effective contributor to the financial success of the organization.

Revenue Cycle Basics

Learning Objectives

- Describe the flow of activities that comprises the revenue cycle of a healthcare facility.
- Distinguish among key players and departments that participate in revenue cycle activities.
- Define the health information management (HIM) role in revenue cycle management.
- Identify the revenue cycle functions that can be supported by HIM professionals.
- Explain key revenue cycle performance measures.
- List performance improvement methodologies that apply to revenue cycle management.

Key Terms

- Accounts receivable (A/R)
- Ambulatory payment classification (APC)
- Bill hold
- Bottom line
- Business record rule
- Case-mix index (CMI)
- Charges
- Claim
- Cost
- Data governance
- Data quality standards
- Denials
- Diagnosis-related group (DRG)
- Discharged, no final bill (DNFB)

- Expense
- Hold
- Information governance
- Internal controls
- *International Classification of Diseases, Tenth Revision, Clinical Modification* (ICD-10-CM)
- *International Classification of Diseases, Tenth Revision, Procedure Coding System* (ICD-10-PCS)
- Lean methodologies
- Medical necessity
- Medicare severity diagnosis-related group (MS-DRG)
- Net operating revenue

- Office of Inspector General (OIG) list of excluded individuals/entities
- Patient access
- Patient registration
- Per diem
- Plan-do-check-act (PDCA)
- Prospective payment system (PPS)
- Revenue
- Revenue cycle
- Six Sigma
- Third-party payer
- Total revenue cycle
- Unbilled
- Value added
- Workflow assessment

To ensure that a provider is paid appropriately for services rendered, efficient and effective processes must be in place to track services, calculate expected reimbursement, and process claims. "Efficient claims processing has a direct impact on the ability of a facility to fund its operations, including paying its bills and meeting payroll obligations. HIM plays a direct role in ensuring efficient claims processing by participating in charge description master review, participating in the analysis and minimization of the accounts receivable totals, and ensuring efficient and accurate coding of records" (Davis 2010, 805). **Accounts receivable (A/R)**, the total sum owed to an organization, generally as a result of services rendered, is an important component of the measurement of various revenue cycle monitors. In the following discussion, assume that all examples and descriptions pertain to healthcare, unless otherwise stated. Although all monetary references are to US dollars, the concepts are generally applicable to any stable monetary standard that can be expressed numerically.

Overview of the Revenue Cycle

Revenue cycle refers to the series of activities that connect the services rendered by a healthcare provider with the methods by which the provider receives compensation for those services. **Revenue** is the sum earned by the provider, measured in dollars. Consider the following somewhat historical example. A patient visits a physician in the physician's office for an examination. The physician records some demographic and clinical information about the patient, performs the examination, and renders whatever treatment or medical advice is necessary. Before leaving the office, the patient is required to pay the co-pay or any co-insurance. The physician takes the payment and deposits it in the bank. Breaking this example down into its component parts, as in figure 1.1, illustrates the revenue cycle as it applies to all healthcare facilities: patient intake, clinical services, charge capture, billing, and collections. Of course, the components of the events described change significantly in the presence of a third-party payer, as we will discuss later in this chapter.

Figure 1.1.   Revenue cycle overview

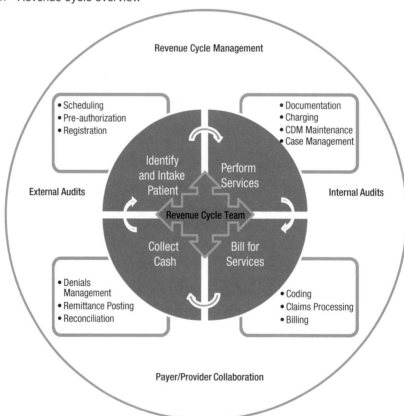

In the hospital setting, the cycle is the same. The hospital also collects demographic and clinical data, treats the patient, sends a bill, and collects the amount due. The fundamental differences in the case of the hospital are in the volume of patients and the types of services rendered. Add the impact of insurance, including case-management governance for average length of stay (ALOS), and other third-party payers, and managing the revenue cycle becomes significantly more complex.

The key players in the hospital revenue cycle are typically whole departments of individuals who support the revenue cycle components. Table 1.1 summarizes the key players and their roles in the revenue cycle. Each of these players has specific issues, concerns, and goals that both inform and depend on efficient and effective revenue cycle management. Subsequent chapters in this text discuss the key players referenced in the following paragraphs in greater detail.

Administration and finance departments look at operational efficiency and effectiveness, achievement of strategic goals, and the maintenance of adequate cash flows to support the business. Payroll, payments to vendors, and investment in and maintenance of the infrastructure are key cash-flow concerns. Managed care, also known as *payer services,* negotiates the payer contracts and the establishment of administrative policies and procedures to ensure accurate reimbursement for services, which are critical components of revenue cycle management.

The patient access department is the data-integrity gatekeeper of the revenue cycle. The data collected and recorded at the point of registration drives many of the controls later in the process; therefore, data quality is the primary concern of this department. Patient access is also responsible for the verification of patients' insurance coverage and precertification or authorization, as needed, of services to be rendered, whereas case management works with the payer to keep the patients medically approved for inpatient services. The HIM department plays a key role in ensuring data integrity and contributes to the revenue cycle in a variety of ways. Again, data quality is paramount. Patient accounting is ultimately responsible for the generation of the bills and

Table 1.1. Key players and their roles in revenue cycle

Department	Roles
Administration	Strategic goals Operational efficiency and effectiveness
Finance	Cash flow
Managed care/payer services	Contract management Material breach issues affecting reimbursement (claims projects)
Patient access	Data integrity and quality assurance Demographic and financial data Insurance verification Precertification
Clinical/ancillary services, including physicians	Documentation of services Documentation and recording of charges
Health information management	Coding Abstracting Data validation and quality assurance
Patient accounting	Compilation of charges Billing Collections

collection of payment. Errors made in other areas flow through to patient accounting, so the timely detection and correction of errors becomes a critical issue.

The financial success of the entire organization depends on each player—including those in clinical services—knowing his or her role and performing the appropriate functions correctly. At some point, each clinical service department is responsible for ensuring that all services rendered are appropriately documented and communicated to patient accounting for billing.

In addition to the key players just discussed, potential players also include case management and information technology. Although case management and information technology are steered in other multidisciplinary committees, their contribution to the revenue cycle should not be underestimated. Case management plays a key role in monitoring length of stay and medical necessity. The capacity and sophistication of information technology drives the facility's ability to control data, monitor their use, and report them intelligently.

Patient Intake

Concomitant with the increasing complexity of healthcare reimbursement in the United States is the greater emphasis on accuracy in collecting and recording patient demographic and financial information. Patients may react cynically when the first question they are asked when encountering the healthcare system is "Do you have insurance?" However, the identification of the means of payment is a key component of the revenue cycle.

Patient access and patient registration are common names for the department that is typically responsible for obtaining the initial demographic and financial information from the patient. (See chapter 4 for an in-depth discussion of the registration function.) Individuals in this department perform what are sometimes called front-end functions, which include but are not limited to the following:

- Recording the reason for visit (admitting diagnosis)
- Verifying and recording patient identifying data, such as name, address, and date of birth. The Social Security number may be collected, but be aware that patients concerned with their privacy and data security may not agree to provide it
- Verifying and recording patient financial data such as insurance and guarantor
- Obtaining precertification/authorization, including submission of the notice of admissions (NOA) for inpatient stays (if required) from the insurer for services to be rendered
- Identifying patients who will need financial assistance to cover the cost of care
- Assigning patient tracking numbers, including the medical record number
- Assigning clinical-service tracking codes, if applicable

Front-end functions take place at the beginning of a process. The provider relies on front-end functions to accurately collect data that will be used later in the process. For example, correct assignment of a medical record number enables the provider organization to link all of a patient's encounters for continuing patient care as well as administrative purposes. Failure to identify a previously assigned number results in the creation of a duplicate medical record number for the patient. Such errors must be corrected later in the process, generally after the patient is discharged. It is easier and less expensive to identify a previously assigned medical record number than it is to research and merge medical record numbers later. From a clinical perspective, failure to identify prior encounters also prevents caregivers from being aware of prior test results and other clinical information. So, correct registration is an important quality of care and patient safety issue. Further, failure to link a current patient encounter with a previous encounter prevents the provider from identifying potential collections issues. In other words, prior balances due will not be identified at registration if the patient's previous relationship with the provider is not linked to the current encounter.

Clinical Services

Once the patient is registered, he or she moves on to the appropriate service area, such as the laboratory, radiology, or same day surgery (SDS). As services are rendered, charges for those services are accumulated. Think of the charge as the description of the service and an associated "retail" price for the service. Providers assign a price to individual charges based on a variety of factors, including cost, payer contracts, and case mix. (Review chapter 5 for a detailed discussion of charges and charge capture.)

There are two front-end activities involved in the provision of clinical services: documenting the service provided and recording the associated charges. From a legal perspective, the medical record falls under the business record rule—that is, the record is admissible as evidence in court, assuming that documentation occurs in the normal course of business and is recorded by authorized, qualified individuals concurrently with the care provided, and that there is no reason to suspect the veracity of the record as presented. As such, the medical record is a long-established means of communication about provider services—if an event is not documented, it is deemed not to have occurred. Similarly, documentation is a critical component of reimbursement. If the service is not documented, or the documentation does not support the charges, the provider is not entitled to payment for that service. The clinical services department plays a lead role in a hospital's ability to meet the requirements of the shared-savings programs discussed in chapter 3, such as Medicare's accountable care organization (ACO), patient-centered medical home (PCMH), delivery system reform incentive program (DSRIP), and value-based purchasing.

Case Management / Utilization Management

The case management department plays a significant role within the revenue cycle process for all inpatient cases. Case management needs to make sure that all managed care patients, whether commercial, managed Medicaid, or managed Medicare, meet the payer's specific utilization management medical-necessity standards. Payers use either the nationally recognized Milliman or Interqual criteria. To be successful at managing inpatient cases for approval by the payers, hospitals are strongly encouraged to invest in a case management system that can directly launch out to both Milliman and Interqual. Even with diagnosis-related group (DRG)–based managed care contracts, case management must receive an initial approval for the patient to be admitted and then needs to manage the case with the clinical services areas to ensure that the patient stays within the accepted average length of stay (ALOS) for the case's working DRG, a methodology that uses diagnosis and procedure data to assign weights to cases with similar resource utilization. Applying this methodology can be challenging when case management knows the patient no longer meets ALOS criteria, but the admitting physician does not want to discharge the patient. Case management also needs to get Medicaid cases certified and must work with families when Medicare or another payer will no longer cover the inpatient stay. This is when self-pay waivers can be used on the inpatient side.

Charge Capture

Along with documentation of services, the clinical services department must also record the charges for those services. Charges are not just for reimbursement; they may also be used for tracking volume as well as inventory. Imagine getting an oil change at an automobile dealership. The mechanic must record the time spent working on the vehicle as well as the number of quarts of oil used and the disposition of the oil that was removed. With that data, the dealership can track how many oil changes each mechanic can do in a day, ensure timely replenishment of oil supplies, and monitor its costs for disposal of hazardous waste.

A similar process of recordkeeping applies in a clinical setting. If a laboratory test is ordered for a hospital inpatient, a charge must be recorded in the patient's account. Timely collection of laboratory charges enables the facility to track these services not just for reimbursement purposes but also to ensure sufficient laboratory staffing and supplies. Furthermore, tracking of charges enables the facility to reconcile the service activities with the cost of providing the service. For example, if the facility charges for 100 doses of morphine in a period, it can reconcile these charges with the number of doses purchased and the number left in the pharmacy's inventory. This process provides an internal control for detecting discrepancies. **Internal controls** are policies and procedures designed to detect, correct, and prevent errors. (See chapter 5 for a detailed discussion of charge capture and internal controls.)

The process of recording the charge varies, depending on the extent of automation. Manual charge tickets may be completed by the clinician and then entered into the financial system later. Alternatively, charges may be captured through an electronic order-entry system. Regardless of the method chosen for a particular clinical service, charges are most accurately and completely captured at the point of care.

Billing

Once the services have been rendered and the encounter has ended (or the patient has been discharged), the payer can be billed. The preparation of the bill (also known as the **claim**) is a patient accounting function. Typically, healthcare organizations do not bill immediately on discharge. There is a waiting period, up to five days for inpatients and up to seven days for outpatients, that allows for reconciling activities versus charges, making corrections as needed, and applying any additional diagnostic and procedural coding. This waiting period is called the **bill hold**.

It is at the point of billing that all of the front-end processes flow together to create a meaningful communication with the payer. Errors in front-end processing can cause billing delays and denials. Failure to correct billing errors on a timely basis can result in reduced payment from the payer or, sometimes, no payment. Therefore, the active processing of claims to correct errors, obtain documentation, and rebill, is a race against the clock. Patient accounting personnel need to be aware of the specific contracts with each payer regarding not only reimbursement terms but also the time frames for claims processing.

Tracking of outstanding patient accounts is an important performance measure. There are several components of tracking:

- Patients who are still being treated—These patients accumulate charges that cannot be billed because their encounter has not ended. Examples include but are not limited to the following:
  - Outpatients with multiple visits spanning more than one day (such as recurring physical therapy visits) whose charges will accumulate over time
  - Outpatients who were admitted on one calendar day and discharged the next (such as emergency department or observation cases)
  - Inpatients who have not been discharged
- Patients whose encounters have ended but for whom a final bill has not been prepared—The specific report that lists these encounters is often called the **discharged, no final bill (DNFB)** or **unbilled** report.
- Final bills that cannot be sent to the payer due to errors—These bills are on **hold** until the errors are corrected. Errors must be corrected in a timely manner to allow for the meeting of timely filing and clean claim requirements. These are concepts discussed further in chapters 5 and 6.
- Bills that have been denied (returned unpaid) from a third-party payer, also called **denials**—A **third-party payer** is an insurance company or entity, other than the patient, with whom the patient has a contractual relationship regarding payment for healthcare services. Denials need to be addressed through a follow-up process involving patient access services (PAS),

clinical services, case management, and patient financial services (PFS); managed care eventually may become involved if the denial is a material breach issue because a payer is not adhering to its own appeals guidelines or the state's appeals guidelines (if they exist in that state). Denials can have such a significant impact on the hospital's bottom line that this function is often outsourced to a vendor or consultant that can spend the time and effort on the follow-up needed to get denials through the appeals process. Ideally, the hospital should be losing no more than 1 percent of its net patient services revenue to denials. Even if a hospital achieves a denial rate of 1 percent or less post appeal, there is still improvement to be made. Additional root-cause analyses need to be done, as is discussed later in this chapter. Furthermore, when an internal department or outsourced vendor achieves a high overturn rate for denials (greater than 60 percent), work needs to be done to determine the root causes of the denied claims because the high overturn rate means something that was "easily" overturned on appeal was missed during the revenue cycle processes before the claim dropped.

Collections

Once the bill has been sent, the healthcare facility or provider expects payment within a specified time period. Some payers, such as Medicare, receive payments on a routine schedule, and claims review over and above automated edits may lag, with reconciliation of amounts due on a periodic basis. Medicare and Medicaid generally pay claims within 14 days of receipt of a clean claim whereas commercial payers pay as quickly as within 30 days of receipt of an electronic clean claim or 45 days of receipt of a paper clean claim. State managed care regulations and the hospital's payer contracts may alter these time frames. Other payers may review every claim in detail before payment and ask for documentation of every charge. Unless they are an exclusive provider for a health maintenance organization (HMO), most providers have contracts with multiple payers. Detailed knowledge of the contracts with each provider enables patient accounting personnel to prioritize their time when reviewing payments received and analyzing expected payments that have not arrived.

Some patients do not have the resources of a third-party payer or may be seeking services for which their third-party payer will not reimburse. Identifying these patients up front helps the provider manage arrangements for payment or guide the patient into counseling for an appropriate government assistance program, such as Medicaid, which is discussed in more detail in chapter 4.

The Revenue Cycle Team

Regardless of patient care setting, a revenue cycle team should be established to reconcile the competing interests of senior leadership that may arise in the reporting structure and to facilitate the development and implementation of shared goals and objectives. This team should be comprised of key administrative, management, and clinical personnel. It should be charged with both the responsibility and the authority to monitor processes and results as well as to direct change. It is the latter objective that is most challenging—hence the need for authority. Common revenue cycle team activities are listed in figure 1.2.

A variety of subcommittees of the revenue cycle team can be formed so that more intensive review, monitoring, or analysis can take place outside of the regular meetings. For example, if an outpatient sleep center is not collecting the revenue expected, or there is another specific revenue cycle situation, a subcommittee of the revenue cycle team known as a financial operations committee may be formed to determine the root cause of that situation. Financial operations committees are especially important at hospitals where each clinical service area is held accountable for both the department's operational budget and its revenue budget. Ideally, a financial operations committee includes the managers and staff of clinical services as well as representatives from

Figure 1.2.   Key revenue cycle team activities

Routine activities:

- Review key performance indicators (KPIs).
- Conduct inquiries into processes that are not meeting benchmarks.
- Monitor denials and clean-claim rates.
- Initiate performance improvement activities as needed.
- Oversee development and implementation of revenue cycle–related processes.

Strategic activities:

- Set benchmarks for KPIs.
- Identify trends in financial data and make recommendations to administration.
- Anticipate the impact of changing regulations, such as implementation of ICD-10-CM/PCS, on the revenue cycle.

the key revenue cycle areas, such as managed care/payer services, patient access, patient financial services and HIM. The committee members meet to review the current processes versus the future process (or processes) that are needed, which may result in updating the process flow chart and creating a formal write-up of the new process(es) so that the clinical service area can begin accurately capturing its reimbursement.

The HIM Perspective

The traditional role of the HIM professional in the revenue cycle is ensuring that proper diagnosis and procedure codes are used for billing. With the advent of the Medicare **prospective payment system (PPS)** in 1983, the coding function became critical in optimizing reimbursement for hospital inpatient services. PPS reimbursement methodologies gained favor with some providers, and some states even mandated PPS. One of the key benefits of the inpatient prospective payment system (IPPS) is the ability to measure hospital performance through the case-mix index. The **case-mix index (CMI)** is a weighted average of the weights of the **diagnosis-related groups (DRGs)** assigned on discharge: one to each case. The DRG is derived from the diagnosis and procedure codes assigned at discharge. In the hospital inpatient setting, the code sets used for this purpose are the *International Classification of Diseases, Tenth Revision, Clinical Modification* (ICD-10-CM) and *International Classification of Diseases, Tenth Revision, Procedure Coding System* (ICD-10-PCS). Table 1.2 illustrates the relationship between the coding, DRG assignment, and CMI. The hospital's Medicare inpatient payment is then calculated based on the provider's inpatient blended rate calculated by Medicare using the hospital's Medicare cost report (discussed in more detail in chapter 2) multiplied by the DRG's specific weighting. Thus, hospitals need accurate clinical documentation from the clinical services departments so HIM can correctly code to the severity of the case (weighting) within the period of the bill hold (the time between discharge and the automatic release of a bill with no defects). A hospital's financial health depends on the accuracy of each department's responsibilities throughout the revenue cycle process.

In the example shown in table 1.2, there is only one case for each DRG, so the simple (arithmetic) average of the three cases yields a CMI of 1.1334 (rounded to match the number of decimal places expressed in the published weights). Table 1.3 shows the same calculation when a DRG has multiple cases.

Table 1.2. Coding, DRG assignment, and CMI

ICD-10-CM/PCS Codes Assigned	Grouped to MS-DRG	2016 MS-DRG Weight
K80.18 Calculus of gallbladder with other cholecystitis without obstruction 0FT44ZZ Resection of gallbladder, percutaneous endoscopic approach BF131ZZ Fluoroscopy of gallbladder and bile ducts using low osmolar contrast	419 LAPAROSCOPIC CHOLECYSTECTOMY W/O C.D.E. W/O CC/MCC	1.2527
J18.9 Pneumonia, unspecified organism N18.6 End stage renal disease Z99.2 Dependence on renal dialysis 5A1D00Z Performance of urinary filtration, single	193 SIMPLE PNEUMONIA & PLEURISY W MCC	1.4256
F13.20 Sedative, hypnotic or anxiolytic dependence, uncomplicated F40.01 Agoraphobia with panic disorder I10 Essential hypertension HZ2ZZZZ Detoxification services for substance abuse treatment	897 ALCOHOL/DRUG ABUSE OR DEPENDENCE W/O REHABILITATION THERAPY W/O MCC	0.7219
	Case-mix index (Arithmetic average of the weights of all the cases listed.)	1.1334

Source: CMS 2016.

In the example shown in table 1.3, there are 36 cases. The frequency of each MS-DRG is multiplied by its MS-DRG weight to obtain that DRG's contribution to case mix. The total of the case weights (53.3143) is divided by the total number of cases to yield the CMI (that is, Total Weight / Total Cases = CMI):

$$CMI = 53.3143 / 36 = 1.4810$$

As Medicare expanded its PPS program to include hospital outpatients, ambulatory surgery, inpatient rehabilitation, and home care, the need for accurate and timely coding grew in these settings. Table 1.4 lists the settings, the Medicare reimbursement system, and the groupers as well as other information for that setting's PPS. HIM professionals need to be knowledgeable about the coding and reimbursement issues for the settings in which they work. This discussion illustrates the depth to which HIM professionals need to understand their settings.

Although some payers follow the Medicare reimbursement model, many do not. Providers and organizations therefore find themselves contracting with multiple individual payers for reimbursement. Coding continues to be an important factor in these contractual arrangements. For example, a payer may reimburse for an inpatient stay based on a **per diem** amount (a fixed daily payment); however, the medical necessity for that stay may be screened on the basis of the coding. **Medical necessity** refers to a set of criteria with which a payer decides what level of care it will reimburse. Theoretically, this same set of criteria drive patient care from the provider's perspective. Chapter 3 explores the relationship between payer and provider in more detail.

While coding may be the most obvious HIM contribution to the revenue cycle, it is certainly not the only one. All of the processes and procedures in the HIM department have the potential to affect the revenue cycle either directly or indirectly.

Table 1.3. Weighted average of case weights determines (CMI)

MS-DRG	MS-DRG Description	# of Cases	MS-DRG Weight	Sum of Case Weights	Case Mix Index
004	TRACH W MV 96+ HRS OR PDX EXC FACE, MOUTH & NECK W/O MAJ O.R.	1	10.9227	10.9227	
064	INTRACRANIAL HEMORRHAGE OR CEREBRAL INFARCTION W MCC	5	1.7317	8.6585	
069	TRANSIENT ISCHEMIA	2	0.7214	1.4428	
093	OTHER DISORDERS OF NERVOUS SYSTEM W/O CC/MCC	1	0.6974	0.6974	
176	PULMONARY EMBOLISM W/O MCC	5	0.9371	4.6855	
193	SIMPLE PNEUMONIA & PLEURISY W MCC	1	1.4256	1.4256	
195	SIMPLE PNEUMONIA & PLEURISY W/O CC/MCC	4	0.7104	2.8416	
243	PERMANENT CARDIAC PACEMAKER IMPLANT W CC	1	2.6550	2.655	
291	HEART FAILURE & SHOCK W MCC	3	1.4822	4.4466	
419	LAPAROSCOPIC CHOLECYSTECTOMY W/O C.D.E. W/O CC/MCC	2	1.2527	2.5054	
621	O.R. PROCEDURES FOR OBESITY W/O CC/MCC	6	1.5469	9.2814	
795	NORMAL NEWBORN	2	0.1758	0.3516	
419	LAPAROSCOPIC CHOLECYSTECTOMY W/O C.D.E. W/O CC/MCC	1	1.2527	1.2527	
193	SIMPLE PNEUMONIA & PLEURISY W MCC	1	1.4256	1.4256	
897	ALCOHOL/DRUG ABUSE OR DEPENDENCE W/O REHABILITATION THERAPY W/O MCC	1	0.7219	0.7219	
Total	Total Weight / Total Cases = CMI 53.3143 / 36 = 1.4810	36		53.3143	1.4810

Source: CMS 2016.

Considerations Within the HIM Department

From the provider's perspective, in a perfect world, a patient record would remain open on the care unit until all clinicians have completed their documentation, regardless of how long that takes. Then, when the record is completed, HIM staff would analyze the data collected in the record, code it slowly and carefully (chatting real-time with physicians and other clinicians, who gladly amend records to clarify any confusing or incomplete documentation), enter the codes, and finalize the completed and coded record with assurance that everything possible has been done to ensure the coding is accurate. If this perfect world included compliance with regulatory and accreditation record completion standards, the process could take up to 30 days postdischarge. Forty years ago, when reimbursement was not tied to coding, this pace of record keeping was not unusual. Although most HIM departments would obtain control of the charts soon after discharge, the coding process was not rushed.

In the current (real world) environment, providers expect to release the account for billing, or "drop a final bill," in less than a week, as noted earlier. Therefore, the focus of the HIM department's process is to obtain control of the chart, code it as quickly as possible, and drop the bill. In this respect, the bill hold drives the process. An aggressive inpatient bill hold requires a bill

Table 1.4.   Medicare PPS overview

Prospective Payment System (PPS)	Acronym	Provider	Brief Summary	Implementation
Diagnosis-related group	DRG	Acute care	More than 700 DRGs. One DRG is assigned per patient stay	October 1, 1983
Medicare severity diagnosis-related group for Inpatient Prospective Payment System (IPPS)	MS-DRG	Acute care	Nearly 999 MS-DRGs; not all numbers are currently assigned to allow for future expansion. One MS-DRG is assigned per patient stay	MS-DRGs transitioned beginning in fiscal year (FY) 2008
Ambulatory payment classification	APC	Ambulatory	More than 700 APCs. It is possible for one patient stay to have more than one APC	August 1, 2000
Resource-based relative value scale	RBRVS	Services covered by Medicare Part B using the Medicare Fee Schedule	Reimbursement for professional services, particularly physicians	January 1, 1992
Resource utilization groups, version III	RUG-III	Skilled nursing facilities (SNFs)	44 or 45 RUGs. Based on Minimum Data Set (MDS) 3.0. Per diem determined by case-mix adjusted payment rates	July 1, 1998
Home health resource group	HHRG	Home health	Groups and weight assigned based on standardized assessment criteria	October 1, 2000
Inpatient psychiatric facility DRGs	IPF PPS DRGs	Inpatient facility	Based on IPPS DRGs; however, the calculation of payment is different	Phased in beginning in FY 2006
Case-mix group for Inpatient Rehabilitation Facility PPS	CMG	Inpatient rehabilitation facility	More than 100 CMGs, based on standardized assessments	Phased in beginning in FY 2002
Medicare severity-adjusted long-term acute care diagnosis related groups	MS-LTC-DRG	Long-term acute care facilities	Corresponds to IPPS MS-DRGs—different weights and lengths of stay	Phased in beginning in FY 2003

drop in three days. There are very few legitimate reasons to hold a bill longer than three days. Examples of plausible delays include dictations pending pathology studies, physician queries, or Medicaid certification. All members of the HIM team need to be aware of and respond appropriately to the urgency created by this driver.

In a paper-based or hybrid record environment, the paper portions of the record must be obtained from the care unit quickly, generally the morning after discharge. The faster the coders receive the chart, the sooner any issues can be identified and addressed. If the coders need to wait for paper portions of the record to be scanned into the document management system, then the timing of the scanning process becomes a critical factor in timely coding. Chapter 6 explores these issues in more detail. Chart completion and release of information are also important because payers will sometimes require documentation of questionable services or patient accounting may need to include documentation to support rebilling of denied claims. So, the HIM department needs to move quickly to identify the components of the discharged record, make the record available to the coders as soon as possible, resolve any documentation issues, and ensure that documentation is provided to payers (on request) in a timely manner—ideally, before the end of the bill hold period.

Beyond the clinical documentation required to code the chart are myriad other inputs that can affect timely billing. For example, accurate registration of the patient is critical to ensuring that the correct payer is billed under the correct policy. While the HIM department is not generally responsible for the financial data collected by patient registration, there are other data, such as sex, that can affect coding and therefore billing. For example, a record for a female patient with a diagnosis of prostate cancer is problematic. The HIM department may also be responsible for coordinating the resolution of potential billing errors regardless of the source of the error. For example, an error in the posting of room and board charges may delay billing until it is resolved. Because multiple departments and functional areas must contribute data toward an accurate bill, the HIM department must collaborate with many other players to be effective.

Partnering with Other Departments

The HIM department needs to partner with other departments to ensure efficient and effective services. Postdischarge processing is essentially a support service because it does not provide direct patient care; therefore, members of the HIM department need to know their customers and provide excellent customer service. To support the revenue cycle, there are three key departments with which HIM needs to partner: patient access, patient accounting, and the medical staff office.

Patient access is at the front end of the revenue cycle, and HIM is in the middle. During the coding and chart completion process, HIM staff will review and validate certain data elements, such as physician identifiers, patient gender, and admitting diagnosis. For quality assurance and improvement purposes, errors in capturing fields such as these must be called to the attention of the patient access department. Correction of some errors may not be possible in HIM and must be referred back to patient access. Thus, HIM performs an essential data-quality internal control function by detecting and correcting front-end errors. Failure to correct these errors may result in delayed billing or claims denials. See chapter 4 for more information on patient access.

Patient accounting is at the back end or, in other words, near the end of the revenue cycle process. By the time patient accounting receives the data, the account is typically at least three days postdischarge, and the time period for the provider to submit an original claim for reimbursement is diminishing. Any errors that remain in the data will either prevent the claim from going through to the payer or may result in a denial of payment from the payer. The creation of a clean (error-free) claim is discussed in detail in chapter 6. HIM and patient access must work closely and efficiently with patient accounting since many of the errors that hold up a bill from processing are either generated by or researched and corrected within these areas. Some providers rely almost entirely on patient accounting to resolve billing errors. However, "depending solely on patient accounting to resolve billing issues, which may often require input from patient access or HIM, does not foster an environment of performance improvement" and errors will continue to occur (Handlon 2015). "Identification, trending, education, and communication are key to successful collaboration of these departments and, in turn, successful submission of claims" (Handlon 2015).

The medical staff office, although not an obvious contributor to the revenue cycle, is nonetheless important because it is the gateway to the physician data. For proper payment, the attending and operating physicians must be identified. If the provider identification is not maintained accurately, bills will be held until the data can be corrected. Further, the medical staff office must ensure that physicians are eligible to bill relevant payers (for example, Medicare and Medicaid). Physicians who are on the Office of Inspector General (OIG) list of excluded individuals/entities cannot bill Medicare (OIG 2015). This exclusion extends to writing orders for tests that a laboratory or hospital would provide. Therefore, failure to properly identify and credential a physician can lead to billing problems for the facility.

Data and Information Governance

Data governance deals with the quality and integrity of data within an organization, wherever and however data are collected, transmitted, and stored. Data governance includes, for example, data quality and security (Johns 2015, xxii–xxiii). According to the 2014 Benchmarking White Paper on Information Governance in Healthcare (Knight and Stainbrook 2014) information governance establishes a "comprehensive platform for the effective and efficient management of the information lifecycle" (Knight and Stainbrook 2014). Information governance does the following:

- Establishes policy-level rules
- Defines investment priorities
- Institutes accountabilities
- Aligns implementation outcomes to business priorities
- Measures results (Knight and Stainbrook 2014)

Information governance, then, speaks to the *use* of data, including release of information and records management. To further distinguish data governance and information governance, think back to the patient access examples previously discussed. Data governance covers what data are collected and how these data are safeguarded. It is concerned with the registrar obtaining and validating patient identification and financial data (that is, insurance or other method of payment). Information governance covers who has access to these data and how they are used; for example, it concerns the release of records to a payer.

The importance of information and data governance in the revenue cycle cannot be overstated. In the rapidly changing reimbursement environment, high-quality analytics for decision-making require data that are timely, accessible, accurate, and relevant. For example, value-based purchasing models require that facilities maintain specific levels of clinical outcomes in order to receive full reimbursement. The ability to track, analyze, and improve clinical outcomes, even in an electronic health record environment, depends on the availability of accurate data. Therefore, the organization must be collecting the data in the first place, in the most useful format, consistently and accurately.

HIM Roles in Revenue Cycle Management

In this chapter, we have been referring to the HIM department as a generic substitute for a wide variety of roles that HIM professionals may play in revenue cycle management. In fact, HIM professionals at all levels may play some role in managing or supporting an efficient and effective revenue cycle. Individuals who are interested in a revenue cycle career path should be competent in reimbursement methodologies, clinical classification systems, project management, and team building. A quick look at the Health Information Career Map (AHIMA 2015) and the HIM academic competencies (see online appendix 1.3) illustrates that HIM professionals are well suited for a revenue cycle career path.

At the entry level, there are billing- and insurance-related jobs such as medical biller, billing customer service, and collections clerk. The entry-level competencies for HIM programs at the associate-degree level cover the work-based skills needed for these positions. For example, graduates of an accredited associate-degree HIM program can apply and evaluate the application of diagnosis and procedure codes appropriate to settings across the continuum of care, analyze current regulations and established guidelines in clinical classification systems, and evaluate revenue cycle management processes. This training also supports midlevel functions such as coding, clinical documentation improvement, and revenue cycle auditing.

At the advanced level, baccalaureate-level training in managing data, implementing processes for revenue cycle management, and reporting and applying principles of healthcare finance for revenue management supports HIM practitioners as managers of coding and the revenue cycle and in related consulting roles. Ultimately, HIM practitioners with additional training in leadership and strategic models can move into administrative roles.

Thus, the broad work-based training that HIM professionals obtain through accredited training programs includes very specific competencies that address revenue cycle management. Therefore, HIM is a logical career path for practitioners with an interest in the revenue cycle.

Check Your Understanding 1.1.

1. Describe the flow of the revenue cycle.

2. How does the medical record relate to the revenue cycle?

3. What is a bill hold, and why is it important in the revenue cycle?

Performance Improvement Issues

The goals for improving revenue cycle performance include but are not limited to improving data quality, producing clean claims, and reducing denial rates. Improved revenue cycle performance is not necessarily about treating more patients or expanding services, although those are certainly reasonable strategies for increasing revenue. Treating more patients does not improve performance if the facility is losing money on every case. Therefore, the purpose of performance improvements is greater financial efficiency when treating the patients you have. On the other hand, if the goal of treating more patients in a particular service were to provide a gateway service that would lead to more reimbursement with subsequent services, the "lost" money from that particular service should be measured against the results as a whole. In this case, a healthcare organization should evaluate whether the loss-leader service yields the desired increase in reimbursed services. For example, does expanding pediatric services at a loss increase the volume of profitable maternity services to the extent that the loss in pediatrics is at least compensated by the increase in maternity service revenue? Thus, performance improvement in the revenue cycle starts in the same place as all other activities, with the identification of the plan, strategic goal, or problem to be solved. Depending on the desired financial outcome, different strategies may be employed, such as dashboards for monitoring KPIs for back-end reporting, discussed in chapter 5. Dashboards give a snapshot of data, such as the day's DNFB and the hospital census (the number of admitted patients at a point in time). They typically have icons, emoticons, or "stoplight" colors that highlight whether a measure is satisfactory (signaled by, for example, a happy face or green highlights), unsatisfactory (a sad face or red highlights), or needs attention (a slight frown or yellow highlights). Figure 1.3 is an example of a dashboard.

Establishing Benchmarks

Typically, the desired outcome of any revenue cycle activity will be related to increasing revenue, accelerating the billing process, and increasing the rate or volume of collections. The roots of the activity lie deep in the data collection and recording processes. These processes are often executed by individuals who have little or no knowledge or understanding of how their activities affect the outcome. There can be negative consequences if a registrar assigns a new medical record number to a patient instead of using the existing one. If this patient is in default of his or her financial obligations to the facility, the collections opportunity is missed because the new medical record number will not be associated with the old, outstanding account. Collection of outstanding debts may not be the main responsibility of the registrar, but it is obvious from this simple example that the revenue cycle touches more than just the PFS department.

There are many ways to monitor revenue cycle performance. Examples of KPIs include the total amount of receivables, cash flow, DNFB, and denials. These measures, which can be benchmarked against similar facilities, loosely fall into the following three categories:

- Optimizing revenue
- Timely billing
- Increasing collections

Benchmarks can be established by reviewing and evaluating professional literature, such as publications from the Healthcare Financial Management Association, as well as published data from hospital associations and private consulting firms. A potential benchmark or threshold for a registrar would be 100 percent accuracy in the capture of previous hospital encounters. Capturing previous encounters is such a critical activity that it might also be tied to both patient access departmental performance and the registrar's individual performance evaluation. Identifying the critical drivers of specific revenue cycle outcomes is a necessary step in the performance improvement process.

None of the revenue cycle performance measures listed is the sole responsibility of any one individual or department in an organization. This point can be discussed from a different perspective by describing the multiple drivers of revenue: market size, market share, product mix, and quality (Cleverley et al. 2011). Thus, to determine the measurement from which performance improvement will be baselined and improved, the critical drivers of the desired measure must be identified.

One key issue in benchmarking is the comparison of data among peer providers—for example, providers of the same size and type. Drilling down to individual department-level performance is helpful, if that data can be obtained. Examples of measures that can be benchmarked include DNFB dollars and outstanding A/R. However, it is more meaningful to benchmark DNFB monies as a percentage of a target dollar amount, such as A/R, than to take into consideration only the DNFB itself. A great example of market data is the Financial Analysis and Statistical Trends (FAST) Report of New Jersey Hospitals, published quarterly by the New Jersey Hospital Association (NJHA). An example of this report is included in the online materials for this text. This type of report provides administration with a quarterly analysis of financial and operational KPI data in a comparative format. The report includes comparative data such as days in A/R and profit and loss per adjusted day, including CMI and ALOS comparisons. In one study, summarized in table 1.5, the authors analyzed DNFB as a percentage of the **total revenue cycle**, which they defined as the sum of the average number of days in DNFB and the average number of days in A/R. This method is more meaningful than merely comparing the dollars in DNFB because it looks at the overall performance rather than a point-in-time measure.

Figure 1.3.   Sample administrative dashboard

2016 AR Dashboard   Meeting Date: 7/5/2016

POS Collections	Goal		Report Date	6/24/2016	Variance from Benchmark	
	$ Amounts	% of Total	$ Amounts	% of Total	$ Amounts	% of Total
Collected at POS			$ 17,456	31.6%		
Unpaid Balance on Notes			$ 27,389	49.6%		
Amount Paid & Balance on Notes	$ 56,000	100.0%	$ 56,879	103.0%	$ 879	
Total Patient Responsibility			$ 55,245	100.0%		
Missed Money	$ -	0.0%	$ 11,263	20.4%		
Total Discharges			1,502			
Accts with Est Resp >$0			287			
Accounts missing Est Resp			198			
Missed $$ / Total Admissions			$7			

Comments
Large shift in the % of non-missed that was put on payment plans as opposed to paid in cash. Need to monitor as third quarter continues to progress to ensure this trend does not continue.

Aged from Discharge Date Gov't Receivables	Benchmark: 12/31/2015 Over 90 days		Report Date 7/4/2016 Over 90 days		Variance from Benchmark Over 90 days	
	Balance	# of Accts	Balance	# of Accts	Balance	# of Accts
Medicare	225,011	270	617,866	748	392,855	478
Medicaid	63,824	95	85,591	165	21,767	70
Tricare	227,264	41	107,925	110	(119,340)	69
TOTAL Governmental	516,099	406	811,381	1,023	295,282	617
Non-Gov't Receivables	Over 90 days		Over 90 days		Over 90 days	
	Balance	# of Accts	Balance	# of Accts	Balance	# of Accts
BCD - Medicare Supplement	30,998	13	15,071	50	(15,926)	37
BCD	137,779	63	61,103	40	(76,676)	(23)
BCD Total	*168,776*	*76*	*76,174*	*90*	*(92,602)*	*14*
UVW - Medicare	-	-	6,370	1	6,370	1
UVW - Medicare Supplement	2,452	7	2,907	18	455	11
UVW	44,950	55	34,082	33	(10,867)	(22)
UVW Total	*47,402*	*62*	*43,360*	*52*	*(4,042)*	*(10)*
MNO - Medicare Supplement	6,671	4	4,249	5	(2,422)	1
MNO - Medicare	28,152	44	31,834	44	3,682	-
MNO - (employee benefits)	16,150	22	1,098	5	(15,052)	(17)
MNO	187,266	51	61,941	43	(125,325)	(8)
MNO Total	*238,240*	*121*	*99,123*	*97*	*(139,117)*	*(24)*
ABC - Medicare Supplement	1,166	12	67,387	11	66,221	(1)
ABC - Medicare	9,827	10	9,399	4	(428)	(6)
ABC - Mediciad	521	2	2,715	2	2,195	-
ABC	59,566	68	20,117	25	(39,449)	(43)
ABC Total	*71,080*	*92*	*99,619*	*42*	*28,539*	*(50)*
WXY - Medicare	46,756	18	17,798	12	(28,958)	(6)
WXY	15,760	3	-	-	(15,760)	(3)
WXY Total	*62,517*	*21*	*17,798*	*12*	*(44,718)*	*(9)*
STU - Medicaid	44,627	48	87,861	95	43,234	47
STU Total	*44,627*	*48*	*87,861*	*95*	*43,234*	*47*
TUV Direct Choice	37,264	32	19,727	10	(17,537)	(22)
TUV Choice Total	*37,264*	*32*	*19,727*	*10*	*(17,537)*	*(22)*
VBH	-	-	330	1	330	1
VBH Total	*-*	*-*	*330*	*1*	*330*	*1*
Other Medicare Supplement	30,670	56	4,468	75	(26,202)	19
Other Managed Medicare	105,315	90	97,465	65	(7,850)	(25)
Other Managed Medicaid	192,811	79	140,362	89	(52,449)	10
Other Commercial	153,697	65	106,407	18	(47,290)	(47)
Other Managed Care	178,643	169	55,945	49	(122,698)	(120)
Workers' Comp	292,837	83	115,462	76	(177,375)	(7)
Other Misc	1,942	11	-	-	(1,942)	(11)
TOTAL Non-Governmental	1,625,820	1,005	964,100	771	(661,720)	(234)
GRAND TOTAL	2,141,919	1,411	1,775,481	1,794	(366,438)	383

Comments
*Total Insurance Receivables is up $329,000 from last week due to completion of ABC claims project worth $250,000.
Plus additional increase of $79,000 from all other payers.*

Governmental Out-of-Period Recoupments (RAC & MIC Audits)	2015	2016 YTD	Month: July	Comments
Medicare	(33,718)	(68,725)	-	
Medicaid	(272,569)	(98,952)	(34,714)	7 accounts recouped in June: 5 O/B and 2 PSY

^Avg 2015 includes data available on prior AR Dashboard. Late Charges and Cash Collected: week ending 6/22/16; Denials: week ending 7/01/16

Figure 1.3. Sample administrative dashboard (Continued)

Late Charges	Benchmark Avg 2015^	Report Date 7/1/2016	Variance from Benchmark
Total Charges > 3 days past DC	$ 154,378	$ (289,706)	$ (444,084)
Total Charges > 3 days past DOS	$ 328,943	$ 203,147	$ (125,796)
Unique Accounts (DOS rule)	257	876	619
Total Lines (DOS rule)	903	2729	1826
Total Quantity (DOS rule)	901	889	(12)

Comments
Negative late charges due to significant charge corrections made to accounts for pharmacy charges for month end processing. Meeting scheduled to discuss how to best move forward with pharmacy charge processes when CDM charges are updated. $58,733 in Professional Fees moved from 401 accounts, but zero sum effect on late charges.

Cash Collected	Weekly Goal	Report Date 7/1/2016	Variance from Benchmark
Insurance		$ 1,810,645	
Patient		$ 90,084	
TelePsych		$ 32,564	
Employee		$ 7,563	
Total	$ 1,897,623	$ 1,940,856	$ 43,233

Comments
Above goal for the week due to large finalizing Managed Care claims projects collections. Posted to accounts on 06/30/2016. Behind goal for the first 4 days of the month by $165,689. July 1st and 2nd had no Medicare collections.

Aged from Date of Last Pt Pmt Or Discharge if no Pmt / Self Pay Receivables	Benchmark: 12/31/15 0 - 30 days	Account Balances %	TOTAL	Report Date 7/4/2016 0 - 30 days	Account Balances %	TOTAL
9000 - No Note	75,466	7.8%	970,537	256,739	11.4%	2,254,255
9001 - Account with ABC	30,361	1.9%	1,632,913	22,486	2.2%	1,038,219
9050 - Note with ABC	270,553	78.2%	346,077	126,752	65.7%	192,960
9080 - Hospital Note	237,558	43.3%	548,799	409,676	37.8%	1,083,461
9020 - Medicaid Pending	-		4,216	-		28,784
Self Pay Packages	55,523	40.6%	136,742	7,064	1.7%	421,705
TOTAL Self Pay	669,460	18.4%	3,639,283	822,718	16.4%	5,019,384
Self Pay Receivables	0 - 30 days	# of Accounts %	TOTAL	0 - 30 days	# of Accounts %	TOTAL
9000 - No Note	175	9.0%	1,934	249	10.2%	2,450
9001 - Account with ABC	48	2.3%	2,103	15	0.9%	1,613
9050 - Note with ABC	90	52.3%	172	28	30.8%	91
9080 - Hospital Note	264	35.6%	741	366	30.1%	1,214
9020 - Medicaid Pending	-		1	-		4
Self Pay Packages	13	50.0%	26	20	9.2%	218
TOTAL Self Pay	590	11.9%	4,977	678	12.1%	5,590

Comments
Self Pay Package Process was discussed. Pending resolution on 9050 and 9080 account clean up.

DNFB by Service Line	Dollars	Days in AR
Med/Surg	$ 2,754,349	2.74
Psych - DT	$ 15,984	0.02
Psych - Spec.	$ 782,231	0.78
Rehab - Spec.	$ 305,597	0.30
Ancillary	$ 592,394	0.59
Imaging	$ 293,276	0.29
Peds Clinic	$ 45,958	0.05
Adult Clinics	$ 63,223	0.06
Closed	$ -	-
Blank	$ -	-
TOTAL	$ 4,853,013	4.83
On Desk*	$ 1,284,105	1.28
* On Desk data is a week behind DNFB data		

Comments
HIMS is working on a plan to reduce overall days in A/R from 4.83 to 3 days based on expected target.

Billing Issues Log	Goal	Report Date 7/4/2016	Variance from Benchmark
Total $ Amount	$ 50,000	$ 327,409	$ 277,409

Comments
Med/Surg $127,203; OBV $43,002; Sleep $37,694; Clinics $22,306; HIM $96,504

Adjustments, Denials, Charity	Benchmark Jan-Jun 2016	Prior Month Jun 2016	Current Month Jul 2016
Past Filing Deadline	$ 8,914	$ 28,410	$ 238
No Auth	$ 28,556	$ 17,897	$ 14,444
Non-Covered Charges	$ 41,957	$ (2,441)	$ 11,831
Late Charge	$ -	$ -	$ -
Professional Courtesy	$ 97	$ 45	$ -
Administrative Writeoff	$ (13,390)	$ 1,630	$ 1,439
Charity Care	$ 61,897	$ 49,306	$ 12,095
TOTAL	$ 128,032	$ 94,847	$ 40,047

Comments
Trending on target for July; have only had to write off 1 account this month.

Denials	Benchmark Avg 2015^	Report Date 6/24/2016	Variance from Benchmark
Collected by Week	$ 85,865	$ 89,994	$ 4,129
Total Collected (as %)	52.0%	74.0%	22.0%
Lost by Week	$ 13,992	$ 5,177	$ (8,815)
Total Lost (as %)	11.3%	17.5%	6.2%
New Denials by Week	$ 125,920	$ 62,514	$ (63,406)
Total Active Denials	$ 2,296,651	$ 1,051,363	$ (1,245,288)
Total Active (as %)	36.7%	8.5%	-28.2%
Denials (net collectible)*	$ 6,256,966	$ 12,411,089	$ 6,154,123
* Only relevant in the calculations of the % Active, % Lost and % Collected			

Comments
Good collection week
Seeing an increase in Sleep and Imaging denials. Payer Services met with Imaging and Sleep management to discuss process improvements to help reduce denials.

	Bad Debt 2015	Bad Debt 2016	Collection Fees 2015	Collection Fees 2016
January	$ 270,694	$ 313,715	$ 14,771	$ 22,360
February	$ 613,608	$ 246,317	$ 8,117	$ 14,576
March	$ 67,436	$ 108,822	$ 5,099	$ 23,085
April	$ 621,708	$ 121,447	$ 5,690	$ 12,775
May	$ 331,964	$ 591,775	$ 14,489	$ 20,528
June	$ 282,580	$ 328,582	$ 14,820	$ 24,590
July	$ 322,542		$ 15,951	
August	$ 285,329		$ 9,203	
September	$ 389,720		$ 10,300	
October	$ 323,252		$ 12,583	
November	$ 425,786		$ 12,643	
December	$ 668,840		$ 11,773	

2015 Avg through June: $364,665
Avg July through Dec: $402,578

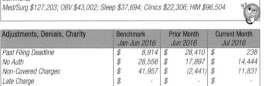

	QA Reports 2015	% at Dschrg	% at Billed
January	77%/90%	85/70/76	98/93/94
February	81%/93%	84/64/71	98/89/93
March	81%/94%	83/53/74	97/85/93
April	83%/93%	83/74/75	97/94/95
May	83%/94%	81/72/73	98/92/94
June	84%/95%	82/73/73	97/93/93
July	85%/96%	81/70/72	96/95/95
August	80%/96%	75/69/69	97/96/96
September	78%/95%	78/70/71	97/91/94
October	78%/94%	82/67/72	95/90/93
November	83%/96%		
December	78%/95%		
	All DC / All Bill	Adm/Cl/Sys	Adm/Cl/Sys

Table 1.5. Benchmarking DNFB at best-performing hospitals

DNFB Compared to Total Revenue Cycle				
Hospital Size	Best Performing Hospitals		Other Performing Hospitals	
	DNFB ≤3 # (%)	DNFB >3 # (%)	DNFB ≤3 # (%)	DNFB >3 # (%)
Small (1–99 beds)	8 (53)	7 (47)	8 (29)	20 (71)
Medium (100–299 beds)	9 (60)	6 (40)	7 (21)	27 (79)
Large (300+ beds)	5 (45)	6 (55)	9 (32)	19 (68)

In half of "best performing" hospitals, DNFB compared to the total revenue cycle is equal to or less than three days.
Source: Amatayakul and Work 2006.

Analysis and Measurement

The *bottom line* means different things to different organizations, depending on the context. For the purpose of this discussion, the **bottom line** is synonymous with **net operating revenue**: operating revenue minus operating expenses. (Refer to chapter 2 for an explanation of accounting terms.) Hospitals have two basic financial strategies to increase their bottom line: increase revenue and decrease costs. Increasing collections (that is, maximizing the percentage of revenue that is actually received) is, of course, important, but collections are reflected more in the balance sheet (cash) than the income statement (net revenue), since the underlying expected revenue based on historical payment calculations has already been recorded, including reserves for possible reimbursement of credit balances to Medicare, Medicaid, or a managed care payer.

Expense is a financial accounting term that reflects the use of resources in a specified period of time, measured in monetary terms. The purchasing of supplies, for example, is recorded as an expense. **Cost** is a management accounting term that refers to the direct or indirect resources used to produce a product or service, either individually or in aggregate. For example, the cost of providing a copy of a record to a patient includes the direct costs of human resources, paper, and photocopier usage as well as the indirect costs of facility space, light, and air conditioning. Additional indirect administrative, housekeeping, and facilities maintenance charges could also be allocated as costs in this example. Paper supplies, then, are expenses when they are purchased, whereas the dollar value of the paper used to copy a record for release is a cost associated with that process. In general, nonaccounting managers tend to use the terms *expense* and *cost* interchangeably when referring to spending that is outpacing the associated revenue stream or targeted budget. The following are the three ways to control costs:

* Daily management of costs
* Process-based cost savings
* Strategic cost management (IMA Consulting 2008)

Daily management of costs refers to the management activities of controlling spending, including supplies and personnel, and ensuring that the various parts of the organization are operating within budget. *Process-based cost savings* ideally yield savings from increased efficiency and effectiveness. *Strategic cost management* is a long-term approach in which goals are set and the organization moves toward those goals. Organizations that combine all three of these cost-control measures are most likely to achieve long-term success (IMA Consulting 2008). The operating and capital budget cycles help codify spending limits, and periodic variance analysis will enable management to identify cost-control problems. However, it is the commitment of the line management and staff to control costs that has the most impact on ensuring financial compliance. When an organization practices strategic cost management, continuous analysis of the relationship between revenue and expenses as well as functional costs will marry the daily cost-control measures with the strategic vision. To look at process-based cost analysis, a complete understanding of the cost contribution of the process to the gross margin is needed. In clinical areas, there is a direct relationship between those costs and the charges (record of individual services performed).

Hospital inpatients accumulate charges during their stay for room and board, pharmacy, laboratory, radiology, and other services. If the payer is Medicare, which reimburses based on **Medicare severity diagnosis-related groups (MS-DRGs)**, those charges are for the most part not connected to the estimation of expected payment. However, identifying charges is critical for evaluating inpatient services as well as identifying cost-to-charge ratios, which are discussed in chapter 2. For many outpatient services, the relationship between charges and payments is clearer: Perform a laboratory test, charge for that test. In both inpatient and outpatient settings, if the coded diagnoses and procedures are not reflected in the charges, the payer will likely deny the claim. Imagine that the claim documents a chest x-ray service with a diagnosis of decubitus ulcer of the foot and a Current Procedural Terminology (CPT) code for an endoscopy. If the billing system is set up to compare services, diagnoses, and codes and flag those that are incompatible, the bill will be held for analysis and correction. If the system cannot do the comparison, the bill will be sent and the claim will be denied. Therefore, accurate, timely, and complete charge capture and coding are essential for efficient reimbursement. This topic is discussed in detail in chapter 5.

Quality Assurance

As described earlier, accurate registration and accurate coding are key drivers of accurate billing. Data quality assurance, then, is a critical activity of the patient access and HIM departments. **Quality assurance** is any activity that verifies the compliance of a process or the output of a process with predetermined standards. For example, a supervisor's check of a registrar's work to make sure that all critical fields are completed is a quality assurance activity. In this case, the supervisor's check is also an internal control activity, as discussed in chapter 4.

Ensuring the quality of data involves the development and implementation of data quality standards. Figure 1.4 details the essential principles of healthcare documentation developed by the Medical Records Institute (2002).

Data quality standards are the specific organization-based rules that define what data are to be collected, how these data will be recorded and edited, and how they will be retained. Organizations tend to follow one of three formal data methodology standards: Plan-Do-Check-Act (PDCA), Six Sigma, or Lean methodologies. *Completeness* is a standard that must be defined by the organization in each instance of data collection. To ensure that the standard of completeness is met, procedures should be developed and implemented to review the data collection systematically for this element. This review is simplified by applying computerized controls at the point of data entry to prevent the user from proceeding if a data element is not entered. For some data fields, such as patient name, this type of control is critical. Even entering "unknown name" is preferable to leaving the field blank because name is a critical retrieval field in the master patient index. In other data fields, such as race and ethnicity, the organization may choose to have the system alert the user that data are incomplete but allow completion of the task, because there may be situations, such as emergent cases, in which the patient is not available to the registrar for observation or query. In the HIM department, completeness of data is evaluated, for example, during quantitative analysis and abstracting.

Quality assurance, then, is a routine, continuous process that is applied to all functions either concurrently or retrospectively. It is based on predetermined standards. These standards may be

Figure 1.4.   Essential principles of healthcare documentation

Unique identification of patient systems, policies, and practices should:

- Provide unique identification of the patient at the time of recording or accessing the information.
- Provide within and across organizations:
  - Simple and easy methods to identify individuals and correct duplicate identities of the same individual.
  - Methods to distinguish among individuals, including those with similar names, birth dates, and other demographic information.
  - Linkages between different identifications of the same individual.

Accuracy systems, policies, and practices should:

- Promote accuracy of information throughout the information capture and report generation processes as well as during its transfer among systems.
- Require review to assure accuracy prior to integration in the patient's record.
- Include a means to append a correction to an authenticated document, without altering the original.
- Require the use of standard terminology so as to diminish misinterpretations.

Completeness systems, policies, and practices should:

- Identify the minimum set of information required to completely describe an incident, observation, or intent.
- Provide means to ensure that the information recorded meets the legal, regulatory, institutional policy, or other requirements required for specific types of reports, e.g., history and physical, operative note.
- Link amendments to the original document, i.e., one should not be able to retrieve an original document without related amendments (or vice versa) or notification that such amendments exist and how to access them.
- Discourage duplication of information.
- Discourage non-relevant and excessive documentation.

Timeliness systems, policies, and practices should:

- Require and facilitate that healthcare documentation be done during or immediately following the event so that:
  - Memory is not diminished or distorted.
  - The information is immediately available for subsequent care and decision making.
- Promote rapid system response time for entry as well as retrievability through:
  - Availability and accessibility of workstations.
  - User-friendly systems and policies that allow for rapid user access.
- Provide for automatic, unalterable time-, date-, and place-stamp of each:
  - Documentation entry, such as dictation, uploading, scanning (original, edits, amendments).
  - Access to the documentation.
  - Transmittal of the documentation.

Interoperability systems, policies, and practices should:

- Provide the highest level of interoperability that is realistically achievable.
- Enable authorized practitioners to capture, share, and report healthcare information from any system, whether paper- or electronic-based.

Figure 1.4. Essential principles of healthcare documentation (Continued)

- Support ways to document healthcare information so that it can be correctly read, integrated, and supplemented within any other system in the same or another organization.

Retrievability (the capability of allowing information to be found efficiently) systems, policies, and practices should:

- Support achievement of a worldwide consensus on the structure of information so that the practitioner can efficiently locate relevant information. This requires the use of standardized titles, formats, templates, and macros, as well as standardized terminology, abbreviations, and coding.
- Enable authorized data searches, indexing, and mining.
- Enable searches with incomplete information, e.g., wild card searches, fuzzy logic searches.

Authentication and accountability systems, policies, and practices should:

- Uniquely identify persons, devices, or systems that create or generate the information and that take responsibility for its accuracy, timeliness, etc.
- Require that all information be attributable to its source (i.e., a person or device).
- Require that unsigned documents be readily recognizable as such.
- Require review of documents prior to authentication. "Signed without review" and similar statements should be discouraged.

Auditability systems, policies, and practices should:

- Allow users to examine basic information elements, such as data fields.
- Audit access and disclosure of protected health information.
- Alert users of errors, inappropriate changes, and potential security breaches.
- Promote use of performance metrics as part of the audit capacity.

Confidentiality and security systems, policies, and practices should:

- Demonstrate adherence to related legislation, regulations, guidelines, and policies throughout the healthcare documentation process.
- Alert the user to potential confidentiality and security breaches.

Source: © Peter Waegemann, Claudia Tessier et al. Medical Records Institute 2002.

derived from regulatory or other external sources, or they may be organization-specific. In terms of the development of standards, some basic guidelines can be applied. The American Health Information Management Association (AHIMA) has published two sets of data quality guidelines, which are included in online appendix 1.1.

Plan-Do-Check-Act

Plan-Do-Check-Act (PDCA) is a performance improvement methodology that serves to improve outcomes through the analysis and amendment of processes. In all areas, when a problem is noted, the root cause of the problem is identified and analyzed, and corrective measures are taken. The corrective action is then monitored for success. This methodology is excellent for application when a problem is known or suspected. It does not inherently reveal unknown problems.

Six Sigma

Six Sigma is a variation on PDCA. The primary variation is that Six Sigma employs statistical analysis to assess problems, both to determine whether there is a defect in a process and to determine whether an improvement has been successful. Six Sigma is difficult to implement because training is expensive and the underlying mathematics are generally beyond the understanding of the individuals who must be guided by the statistical output. Six Sigma can be most successfully applied to healthcare when it is used in conjunction with Lean methodologies.

Lean Methodologies

Lean methodologies target waste and inefficiencies in a process in order to streamline the process itself. In an article on using the lean toolbox in healthcare, Thomas Zidel gives examples of seven areas of waste, which fall into the categories of delay, overprocessing, inventory, transportation, motion, overproducing, and defects (Zidel 2006). While all areas of the revenue cycle could potentially benefit from streamlining, two obvious targets are charge capture and patient data capture. Some of the tools and techniques associated with Lean methodologies are listed in figure 1.5. A key component of Lean methodologies is the concept of **value added**. For any process, there is a desired outcome. Any component of the process that contributes positively to the desired outcome adds value. Any component that does not contribute value is waste with respect to that process. Waste can also be viewed in terms of information (redundant data collection and incompatible systems), process (rework and waiting), and physical environment (safety issues, excessive movement, and lack of training (Campbell 2009). However waste is defined, the goal of Lean methodologies is to investigate how to improve performance through streamlining processes.

Figure 1.5. Lean methodology techniques

- Five "whys"—In this technique, simply ask "why" in every situation until you discover the root cause of the problem. Usually, "why" is asked approximately five times before the root cause is identified.

- Five S's (sort, straighten, scrub, standardize, and sustain)—This method, simply stated, is house-keeping.
  - Sort—Get rid of everything that is not used or expected to be used.
  - Straighten—Organize what is kept, have a place for everything, and keep everything in its place.
  - Scrub—Clean the area.
  - Standardize—Establish procedures to keep the area organized.
  - Sustain—Maintain the gains and avoid backsliding.

- Visual controls—This method creates a workplace where everything that is needed is displayed and immediately available. There are four levels of visual controls:
  - Visual indicator—Something that just informs, such as a sign on a patient's door with special instructions.
  - Visual signal—An alert or alarm, such as a nurse call light.
  - Visual control—A mechanism to control behavior, such as a needle box that automatically closes when full to eliminate the risk of overfilling.
  - Visual guarantee—A mechanism that allows only a correct response, such as a medication-dispensing machine that will not dispense a medication without a verification of proper identifiers. A visual guarantee is foolproof.

Source: Oachs 2016, 821.

Workflow Assessment

One set of tools that is useful regardless of the chosen quality or performance methodology is **workflow assessment**, which identifies inefficiencies in a process or system. Volume, quality, and value are key workflow assessment measures. For example, an employee greeter in a patient registration area does not necessarily improve registration efficiency. Patients could be asked to take a number and would then be registered in the order in which they arrived. In many physician offices, a sign-in sheet serves this purpose. However, in a busy hospital setting, where patients do not necessarily enter the facility through the optimum point of entry for the desired service, a greeter adds value by directing patient flow, helping to reduce patient anxiety, and supporting the registration process as needed.

Workflow assessment should be practiced on a regular basis throughout the organization. As with job descriptions, any change in a policy or related procedure should prompt an assessment of how that change affects workflow. An excellent overview of work design and process improvement can be found in chapter 25 of *Health Information Management: Concepts, Principles, and Practice* (Oachs 2016).

International Organization for Standardization

The **International Organization for Standardization (ISO)** is an accrediting body similar to the Joint Commission. It promulgates standards for a variety of industries and practices. Organizations voluntarily comply with ISO standards and obtain certification of that compliance to facilitate trade with other organizations. ISO 9000 guidelines for healthcare were published in 2001 and updated in 2006.

The need for internationally recognized standards arose in the late 20th century because individual organizations could not adequately assess the quality of products and processes originating in other countries. The proliferation of international trade, with sometimes unsatisfactory results, left significant uncertainty in the business community. Spurred by the European Economic Community, the ISO was founded in 1987. Benchmarking to ISO standards is useful for organizations to measure quality, and certification to specific standards is essential in international trade in some industries.

Special Considerations for Specific Practice Settings

The general revenue cycle overview discussed in this chapter is not setting-dependent. Workflow must be designed to facilitate patient care; capture demographic, financial, and clinical data; produce a bill; and collect the reimbursement. For the purpose of this overview, the differences among practice settings are related largely to the volume and complexity of the patients seen and services offered.

Inpatient Settings

In an inpatient setting, the revenue cycle challenge is generally related to the decentralization of control over the components of the cycle. Patient access, patient accounting, and HIM may not report to the same senior leadership. Clinical services, where charge capture and documentation occur, have diverse reporting lines for nursing, medical staff, and ancillary services. Therefore, outpatient services that are attached to and administered through a hospital will have challenges similar to those faced in the inpatient setting.

Outpatient Settings

The complexity of outpatient settings can be in direct proportion to the size and diversity of the facility. Because all registration, insurance-verification, and charge-capture tasks fall to a limited number of employees, it may be a challenge to keep up with administrative tasks. In particular, third-party payers often will only pay for medically necessary services. Therefore, payer-specific lists of medical-necessity requirements may help staff reduce the number of denied claims. The establishment of a PFS manager who is trained in revenue cycle management specific to the setting can be effective in ensuring optimized revenue and faster billing, thereby increasing collections for the provider.

Physician Practices

As with outpatient settings, the challenges of revenue cycle management in a physician practice are directly related to size and diversity of practice. A solo physician can effectively manage the revenue cycle for his or her entire practice if he or she is willing to learn various financial concepts such as data capture and billing processes. However, many physicians use billing services because the billing process is time consuming and generally not a good use of the physician's time—particularly in a busy practice. As the practice grows, or in a multi-physician practice, a business manager can be a good investment.

Check Your Understanding 1.2.

1. Identify revenue cycle functions that can be supported by HIM professionals.

2. Explain key revenue cycle performance measures.

3. List performance improvement methodologies that apply to revenue cycle management.

References

42 CFR 412.160

Amatayakul, M. and M. Work. 2006. Benchmarking RCM: Best practices to enhance the HIM role in revenue cycle management. *Journal of AHIMA* 77(3):46–49.

American Health Information Management Association (AHIMA). 2015. Health Information Career Map. http://www.hicareers.com/CareerMap/.

Campbell, R.J. 2009. Thinking lean in healthcare. *Journal of AHIMA* 80(6):40–43.

Centers for Medicare and Medicaid Services (CMS). 2016. Hospital Inpatient Prospective Payment System (IPPS) Proposed Rule FY 2016, Table 5 (MS-DRGv32 Definitions Manual). https://www.cms.gov /Medicare/Medicare-Fee-for-Service-Payment/AcuteInpatientPPS/FY2016-IPPS-Final-Rule-Home -Page.html.

Cleverley, W.O, P.H. Song, and J.O. Cleverley. 2011. *Essentials of Health Care Finance,* 7th ed. Sudbury, MA: Jones and Bartlett.

Davis, N. 2010. Financial management. Chapter 25 in *Health Information Management: Concepts, Principles, and Practice,* 3rd ed. Edited by K.M LaTour and S. Eichenwald Maki. Chicago: AHIMA.

Handlon, L. 2015. Correspondence with authors. November 17, 2015.

IMA Consulting. 2008. Three-pronged approach to managing hospital costs. *IMA Insights* 6(2). http://www .ima-consulting.com/wp-content/uploads/2014/07/insights-0208.pdf.

Johns, M. 2015. *Enterprise Health Information Management and Data Governance.* Chicago: AHIMA.

Knight, K. and C. Stainbrook. 2014. Benchmarking White Paper: 2014 Information Governance in Healthcare. Minneapolis, MN and Chicago, IL: Cohasset Associates and the American Health Information Management Association.

Medical Records Institute. 2002. Healthcare documentation: A report on information capture and report generation. Consensus Workgroup on Health Information Capture and Report Generation. C.P. Waegemann, C. Tessier, A. Barbash, B.H. Blumenfeld, J. Borden, R.M. Brinson Jr., T. Cooper, P.L. Elkin, J.M. Fitzmaurice, S. Helbig, K. Milholland Hunter, B. Hurley, B. Jackson, J.M. Maisel, D. Mohr, K. Rockel, J.H. Schneider, T. Sullivan, and J. Weber. http://citeseerx.ist.psu.edu/viewdoc/download?doi =10.1.1.467.84&rep=rep1&type=pdf.

Office of Inspector General (OIG), US Department of Health and Human Services. 2015. Exclusions FAQ. https://oig.hhs.gov/faqs/exclusions-faq.asp.

Zidel, T.G. 2006. Quality toolbox: A lean toolbox—using lean principles and techniques in healthcare. *Journal for Healthcare Quality:* web exclusive: W1-7–W1-15. https://www.leanhospitals.org/downloads /JanFeb06.pdf.

Additional Resources

Casto, A.B., and E. Forrestal. 2015. *Principles of Healthcare Reimbursement*, 5th ed. Chicago: AHIMA.

Oachs, P.K. 2016. Work design and process improvement. Chapter 25 in *Health Information Management: Concepts, Principles, and Practice,* 5th ed. Edited by P. Oachs and A. Watters. Chicago: AHIMA.

Financial Basics

Learning Objectives

- List and describe the components of a financial transaction.
- Differentiate among the categories of financial accounts.
- Demonstrate the impact of a financial transaction on the accounting equation.
- Review a simple financial statement.
- Explain the relationship between charges and revenue.
- Distinguish between cost and expense.
- Compare and contrast cost-analysis methods.

Key Terms

- Accounts payable
- Activity-based costing (ABC)
- Asset
- Balance sheet
- Bond covenants
- Cash
- Controllable costs
- Cost allocation
- Cost driver
- Cost object
- Credit line
- Debt
- Direct costs

- Equity
- Fixed costs
- Group purchasing contracts
- Income statement
- Indirect costs
- Inventory
- Liability
- Mortgage
- Net income
- Net loss
- Net profit
- Notes payable
- Overhead costs

- Patient service revenue
- Preferred stocks
- Reserves
- Secured credit
- Standard cost profile (SCP)
- Standard treatment protocol (STP)
- Statement of retained earnings
- Step-down allocation method
- Stock
- Uncontrollable costs
- Unsecured credit
- Variable costs

The services that patients receive must be tracked. Departments need to know how many procedures were performed, what supplies were used, and which patients were seen. Patient accounting needs to know how much to bill the patient or other payer. The payer wants to know whether the services rendered match what was authorized or otherwise payable. Consequently, a detailed list of services and charges must be accumulated in the account. The accounting department wants to know how much net revenue was generated. To determine the amount of net revenue, we have to show how charges become revenue and how the costs associated with delivering those services become expenses.

Sources of Financial Data

Financial records originate with transactions, the smallest component of financial activity. Whereas health records are built from individual data entries, financial reports are developed by cumulating transactions. In this section, we will describe transactions and how they affect the accounting equation around which financial reports are constructed.

Transactions

Financial transactions consist of three fundamental steps: goods and services are provided, the transaction is recorded, and compensation is received. A physician office visit is an easy example of a financial transaction. The physician meets with the patient and conducts an examination. The service provided is an office visit. In the patient's electronic health record (EHR), the physician records the examination and any relevant diagnosis, which generates an evaluation and management (E/M) code that describes the visit. The E/M code represents the charge for the transaction. This E/M code is transmitted to the payer on the claim. The payer approves the claim and remits payment to the physician. Table 2.1 shows the preceding example in steps.

In general, clinical services provided by the healthcare organization make up the bulk of that organization's transactions. The posting of a charge is only one side of the patient account transaction. The system of recording financial transactions is based on balancing the purpose of the transactions with their impact on the organization. The impact of a charge on an organization is an account receivable (A/R), an amount owed to the organization from another entity for goods or services provided; someone will theoretically submit an associated payment for the charge. Charges represent a large number of transactions, but many other types of transactions occur. For example, a facility purchases drugs with the purpose of ensuring that a sufficient and appropriate supply is on hand to treat patients. The purchase of the drugs increases the facility's pharmaceutical **inventory**, the amount of supplies on hand to provide services. The impact of that purchase is the outlay of **cash**, which is defined as money or other assets that can be converted to cash quickly. After the cash is spent on drugs, it cannot be spent on something else. Recording both the increase in inventory and the outlay of cash enables the organization to understand and communicate information about its transactions. The theoretical and arithmetic foundation for the recording of transactions is known as the accounting equation: Assets – Liabilities = Equity.

- **Asset:** Something that is owned or due to be received. In a financial transaction, the compensation that has been earned by providing goods or services generally becomes an asset

Table 2.1.   Steps in a financial transaction

Step	Examples
1. Goods or services are provided.	<ul><li>Physician examines a patient</li><li>Medication is ordered and administered</li><li>Radiology exam is ordered and performed</li></ul>
2. A transaction is recorded.	The charge (date of service, description of the service, and the dollar amount assigned to the service by the organization) is linked to the patient account.
3. Compensation is remitted.	The responsible party (or parties), such as a third-party payer or the patient, pays the amount due for the service.

as soon as it has been earned. Examples of assets include cash, inventory, A/R, buildings, and equipment.

- **Liability:** Essentially a debt. Liabilities are amounts that are owed, often due to the acquisition of an asset. A mortgage is a type of liability. Accounts payable and loans payable are also examples of liabilities.
- **Equity:** The arithmetic difference between assets and liabilities; also called *owner's equity*. In a not-for-profit environment, the difference between assets and liabilities is referred to as the fund balance or just net assets.

The purchase of a computerized tomography (CT) scanner illustrates the accounting equation. The purchase of an expensive piece of equipment is often accomplished by the organization making a cash payment and taking out a loan to pay the balance to the seller (a transaction similar to a consumer buying a car). The CT scanner is an asset whose value is recorded at the price that was paid at the time of the purchase. The loan is a liability. As loan payments are made, the amount owed declines. The initial cash payment is the owner's equity in the scanner. As loan payments are made, the amount of owner's equity in the asset increases.

To use another example, Dr. Silvio purchases a customized van for making home visits in the community. She purchases the van for $100,000, making a down payment (or deposit) of $20,000 and assuming a loan of $80,000. As the loan is paid over five years, the historical value of the van remains the same, the amount of the loan decreases, and Dr. Silvio's equity in the van increases. When the van is completely paid off, Dr. Silvio's equity in the van theoretically equals the historical value of the van.

The other side of a "charge" is patient service revenue. During a patient's encounter with a healthcare provider, the provider performs individual services, and the patient incurs the associated charges. Each charge is recorded in the patient account. Although each completed service provided to the patient (charge) is an individual transaction, the discharge of the patient triggers the functional completion of the transactions and the final bill is recorded as A/R and revenue. Revenue increases the equity, also called *fund balance*. For example, here is the equation as we post the account for a discharged patient with charges of $5,500:

Assets	–	Liabilities	=	Equity
A/R $5,500				Revenue $5,500

The equation balances because both sides of the transaction are posted—the amount that the payer owes (A/R) and the amount that increases revenue (patient service revenue [PSR]). However, the payer is unlikely to remit the full amount of the charges because the payer typically has a contract or other agreement with the healthcare provider to pay some amount less than charges. Therefore, it is important to record receivables and revenue in a way that shows the receipt amount that is expected—the net revenue or the amount of PSR *after* contractual adjustments (CA).

Assets	–	Liabilities	=	Equity
A/R $5,500				PSR $5,500
A/R ($4,000)				CA ($4,000)

Until the final bill is dropped, the account (although technically A/R) is often not formally recorded. Therefore, a list of accounts that have been discharged, not final billed (DNFB) is a critical tool in revenue cycle management. This DNFB list must be reviewed daily and problems solved quickly so that final bills can be dropped in a timely manner.

When the payer remits the reimbursement, it increases cash. Remember that cash includes monetary instruments as well as those instruments that can be converted into cash quickly. The latter are often referred to as *cash equivalents*. For accounting purposes, currency and funds in bank accounts are both considered cash. At the point of sale, such as purchasing lunch in the cafeteria, currency may be tendered. The Centers for Medicare and Medicaid Services (CMS), on the other hand, does not deliver reimbursement to a hospital in truckloads of currency; instead, it electronically transfers funds between financial institutions. Nevertheless, both are considered cash to the hospital. Cash is only recorded, and becomes an asset, when it has been received. Here is what happens to the equation when the cash is received:

Assets	–	Liabilities	=	Equity
A/R $5,500				PSR $5,500
A/R ($4,000)				CA ($4,000)
A/R ($1,500)				
Cash $1,500				

Notice in this transaction had no impact on equity. We recorded the revenue, net of contractual adjustments, when it was earned—effectively, when the patient was billed. Unless there are additional adjustments, the revenue is final. Notice that when the reimbursement is recorded, A/R is reduced by $1,500 and cash is increased by the same amount. At this point, the balance in A/R is zero, but there is no change in the equation, just a change in which asset account holds the dollar amount. There are scenarios in which the amount due from the payer is not fully paid. The topic of collections is discussed in more detail in chapter 7.

Impact of Accounts Receivable on Cash Flow

A/R represents a current asset. If there are delays in processing claims, those receivables will "age"—that is, get farther away from the discharge date. Aged receivables can negatively affect a facility's ability to borrow money if the lender perceives that older receivables have less of a chance of being collected and therefore the organization will have less ability to repay a loan. Failure to claim and collect receivables on a timely basis means that cash comes in slowly and the facility may not be able to keep up with payments on its current liabilities, the largest of which is payroll. Therefore, in a facility for which reimbursement is the largest revenue item and payroll is the largest expense, there is a direct relationship between getting reimbursed and paying employees. Thus, effective revenue cycle management is the concern of every employee, regardless of their direct involvement in revenue cycle activities.

Major Categories of Financial Accounts

Of course, financial transactions are not reported in a table such as those shown in this discussion. The accounting equation is represented by a report called a *balance sheet* or *statement of financial position*. The increase or decrease in equity is reported separately in an *income statement* or *statement of operations*. Before proceeding to review of those statements, it is important to understand the other types of accounts that are included in each of the components of the accounting equation.

Assets

As stated earlier, assets are items owned or amounts due to be received. The organization owns its cash, and A/R is an amount that is due from another entity. Cash and A/R are known as short-term assets because they can be converted to cash quickly or, in the case of A/R, will be collected within one year of posting. Long-term assets include buildings and equipment. Long-term assets are so named because their useful life extends beyond a year and often for many years.

Inventory

An organization has **inventory** if it maintains goods on hand that it intends to sell to a client. IV bags, for example, are part of a hospital's clinical supply inventory because they are on hand to be used to administer therapeutic substances to patients. It is important to distinguish between goods that are available for sale (to be charged to patient accounts) and goods that are used by the organization in other ways. Photocopy paper is inventory for an office supply store. To the hospital, it is used for general business purposes and is considered a *supply,* which is an expense rather than inventory. Hospital inventory includes pharmaceuticals and surgical supplies, such as catheters. Many items used to treat patients have expiration dates; therefore, large inventories of those items would not be maintained but would rather be ordered on an as-needed basis.

Accounts Receivable

A/R is the amounts due from various customers (in this case, patients or payers) or other entities. A/R is a current asset because it is expected that all amounts will be collected within a year of being owed. Tracking and following up on A/R from patient services is a key function of patient financial services (PFS) and a focus of the revenue cycle team. For reporting purposes, A/R is not valued solely on the basis of the charges minus contractual allowances. Instead, the reported A/R value is based on a historical review of what percentage of expected A/R is actually received from the payers. This amount could be significantly less than the posted value, due to denials and other factors that are discussed in chapters 6 and 7.

Liabilities

As previously noted, liabilities are debts, or amounts owed. If we purchase inventory on credit and pay later, we post the dollar amount of the inventory to the inventory asset account and that same dollar amount to a liability called *accounts payable.*

Accounts Payable

Accounts payable is a liability that is created when the organization has received goods or services but has not yet remitted the compensation. Referring to the accounts receivable discussion, the provider of the goods and services records a receivable when payment is not received at the point of the sale. On the other side of that transaction is the organization for which the goods and services were provided. When the recipient of the goods and services does not pay immediately, the recipient records the amount as an account payable. The recipient also records either the acquisition of an asset or the recognition of an expense.

Notes Payable

A *note* is a financial obligation that has specific terms of payment in the form of a contract. Effectively, a note is a type of loan and the liability is **notes payable**. The purchase of high-dollar-value goods or services, such as the earlier CT scanner example, may require a loan (also called a note). In the CT scanner example, the scanner itself is collateral for the note. In other words, if the hospital does not repay the note on a timely basis, the purchase contract could specify that the lender can take possession of the scanner.

Equity

Equity is the arithmetic difference between assets and liabilities. In a for-profit organization, equity is the value of the ownership in the organization. In a not-for-profit organization, equity is known as the fund balance. Conceptually, equity is the net worth of the organization if all of the assets were liquidated and all of the liabilities resolved at their current reported value. At the end of every fiscal year, the balance of revenue versus expenses is calculated, and the difference is added to or subtracted from the owner's equity or fund balance account.

Revenue

Revenue consists of known amounts of earnings. It is the compensation that has been earned by providing goods and services to the client or patient as well as amounts received or earned from other sources. Revenue represents an increase in net assets or fund balance and is reported on a separate statement called the *income statement.*

Patient service revenue, which is the revenue from treating patients, is typically the main source of revenue for a healthcare facility. Indeed, depending on the nature of the facility, patient services may be its only source of revenue. Patient service revenue is typically reported as the net of posted charges and contractual allowances, minus historical allowance for recoupments. Examples of nonclinical services that may generate revenue include employee food services, donated services, monetary donations, and copy fees.

Revenue is typically described by its source. Patient services revenue is considered operating revenue because it is the result of the main activity performed by the organization. Additionally, an organization may have nonoperating revenue from interest on investments. A healthcare organization that generates large amounts of income from investments, possibly as a result of a large endowment fund, may also categorize a small stream of donations and related investment income separately as nonoperating revenue. By contrast, an organization that raises funds in order to provide free care would consider donations to be operating revenue.

The health information management (HIM) department may have some cash flow in from release of information activities. However, this is not truly revenue because it is a reimbursement of the cost of providing copies.

Expenses

Revenue is rarely generated without any reduction of cash or liability being incurred. Organizations have operating and non operating expenses, which correspond to the same types of revenue. Expenses represent a reduction in net assets or fund balance and are reported on the income statement. An expense is an outlay of cash or other reduction in an asset that is attributable to a specific time period. A healthcare facility's electric bill, salaries to employees, and copy machine rental are all expenses in the period in which the obligation was incurred. For example, employees of an institution whose fiscal year ends on December 31 might receive a payroll check on January 8 while the expense of their salaries (along with the associated tax and benefit obligations) was recorded by the employer in the prior fiscal year during which it was earned.

Reserves

In a for-profit organization, the shareholders are covered in the equity section of the balance sheet as owning shares, which have a specific dollar amount assigned to them, typically from the owner's share of the excess of revenue over expenses. However, some amounts are not distributed to the owners; they are retained in the business for anticipated obligations, such as replacement of buildings and equipment. The amounts that are set aside and not distributed to the owners are called reserves. In a not-for-profit organization, reserves are a portion of the fund balance that is set aside for the same purpose. For example, reserves may be earmarked for the resolution of bad debt or to otherwise assist with cash flow.

Reserves are also calculated to hold assets if an audit request has been made or based on historical review of payer recoupments—whether they are cost report based or contract-build errors on the payer's part—and accounts with credit balances on them. PFS may not have identified a pattern in the overpayments, and finance must therefore calculate a reserve based on historical payer recoupments and the CMS cost report or other recoupments. This calculated reserve is a key piece to determining the net patient-revenue value reported on the financial statements to the board of directors or trustees.

Other Financial Management Issues

Among the many issues that affect the revenue cycle are payroll obligations, vendor contracts, financing, and credit. These topics are surveyed in the following sections of this chapter. (Of course, there are many more financial management issues that are relevant in HIM. For greater coverage of financial and accounting issues, the authors recommend *Principles of Finance for Health Information and Informatics Professionals,* which is listed in the resources at the end of the chapter.)

Payroll Obligations

By far the largest cash-flow obligation in the hospital setting is payroll. The cost of human resources may exceed 50 percent of a hospital's total expenses in any period. Employees are an organization's first priority in determining cash needs. Payroll and the expenses of associated benefits are a combination of fixed and variable costs. Such expenses for full-time employees are primarily fixed costs. Expenses for per diem and part-time employees are variable, as their hours depend on volume.

The need to meet payroll obligations is critical in estimating cash flow. Although the connection is not often emphasized in organizations, an organization's ability to make payroll is directly linked to the capture of all charges for services rendered and the preparation and submission of clean claims. Figure 2.1 illustrates this relationship. If a healthcare facility delivers $2 million of services but only collects $1.5 million, that is potential cash lost. If the claims on a $1.5 million account contain errors and will not be accepted by the payer, no cash will return to the facility. This idea is not an esoteric, theoretical, or philosophical principle; it is an economic reality. Therefore, role-based training for all employees regarding their contribution to the revenue cycle is essential.

Figure 2.1. Linking charge capture (cash) to payroll

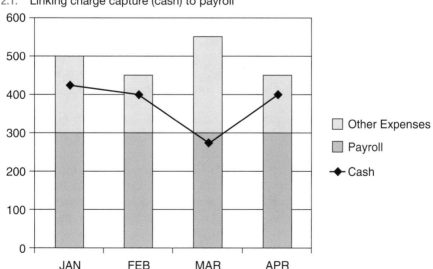

In the example shown in figure 2.1, the healthcare facility consistently receives less cash than is needed to meet expenses. In March, payroll expenses were not covered. The facility had $1.9 million in total expenses for the four-month period but received only $1.5 million in cash during the same period. This healthcare facility must borrow funds or draw down from reserves to pay some of its bills. Although expensive, this sort of situation is not entirely unusual for short periods of time. The revenue earned during the same period may actually be sufficient; however, there is clearly a cash shortage. The administration will likely need to address revenue cycle issues to turn this situation around.

Vendor Contracts

Supplies and services are required to provide patient care, and the number of vendors contracted by an organization to provide those supplies and services can be staggering. Some healthcare organizations may choose to participate in **group purchasing contracts**, such as those offered through some hospital associations. These group contracts enable the healthcare facility to take advantage of discounts offered to larger purchasers. The selection and negotiation of contracts with preferred vendors can also yield considerable cost savings. Centralizing the purchasing function is another way to obtain control over purchasing activities and therefore control cash flow.

If the healthcare organization is in the enviable situation of having sufficient cash to cover all current and long-term obligations on a timely basis, its primary problem will be the appropriate investment of short-term cash. The healthcare facility may also be able to initiate long-term capital investment strategies, such as building infrastructure, obtaining sophisticated technology, and expanding services. However, if outstanding obligations are predicted to exceed the cash on hand, other sources of cash must be explored.

Financing

Depending on the organization's ownership and tax status (for-profit, not-for-profit, or governmental entity), there are a variety of different ways to fund infrastructure and other long-term projects. To finance a building project, for example, the organization may seek debt financing.

Debt is incurred when money is borrowed and must eventually be repaid. A **mortgage** is a type of debt financing. The organization owns the building or other property, but the lender has a secured interest in the property that ensures the money will be repaid. A mortgage is typically repaid in periodic payments, which include interest on the outstanding balance and a portion of the original loan. Another way to finance debt is to issue debt securities, such as notes, bonds, and commercial paper. These instruments have two components: *principal*, which is the outstanding amount of the loan, and *interest*, which may be due periodically or in a lump sum when the debt security expires. Debt financing affects cash flow when there are periodic interest payments due on the principal, or when the instrument expires or becomes payable in full. Some organizations issue new securities when the old ones expire, thus maintaining continuous liability.

Equity securities are shares (**stock**) in the ownership of the organization. Stocks can only be issued by organizations that are permitted to do so by virtue of their tax status, articles of incorporation, and governing body's actions. Not-for-profit organizations and governmental entities are not permitted to sell ownership shares. Ownership of an organization may be closely held, such as family-owned businesses, or shares may be publicly traded on a stock exchange, such as the New York Stock Exchange. Issuance of stock increases cash without creating a liability for repayment. Since shareholders are, effectively, owners of the corporation, they do not expect repayment of the investment. Shareholders participate in the success of the corporation when the governing body elects to distribute dividends or the expectation of corporate success causes the value of the stock to rise. Equity securities affect cash flow if a dividend is declared.

With the exception of certain **preferred stocks**, which have a stated dividend rate, a dividend would normally only be declared if the organization's bottom line permitted doing so without harming the ability of the organization to continue its activities.

Credit

One way to bridge a cash-flow shortage is to obtain a credit line. A **credit line** is a loan that permits the provider to borrow on an as-needed basis and repay as cash is available. Organizations maintain credit lines to support their needs when reimbursement cash received does not meet the immediate cash disbursement obligations. For example, some healthcare organizations that anticipated slower coding, billing, and claims adjudication after ICD-10 implementation obtained or increased lines of credit to bridge the gap until the process settled. If an organization has cash shortages over an extended period of time, the lender may extend the credit line or cut it off, depending on the circumstances.

A credit line may be unsecured or secured. **Unsecured credit** is similar to a retail credit card. Credit is extended based on the overall financial health of the organization and on its credit rating. Similar to the credit rating on individual persons, an organization's credit rating is based on its historical financial performance, current activities, and projected ability to repay over time. A homeowner equity loan is a retail example of **secured credit**—a loan that is based on the value of an *asset* that is owned by the creditor. Examples of assets that might secure a credit line include, but are not limited to, A/R, equipment, inventory, and buildings.

Hospitals have the option to sell bonds to obtain funding. Bonds are debt instruments that may be sold either in a limited market or in the public market. The interest rate on the bond issuance is tied to the market rate at the time of issuance as well as the issuer's creditworthiness. An organization's creditworthiness for this purpose is determined by objective analysis, usually by an external organization such as Moody's. The terms of the bond issuance, called **bond covenants**, are monitored by the external organization, and failure to comply with the terms may negatively affect the hospital's credit rating and, therefore, its ability to borrow in this or any other market. Therefore, the collection of A/R and the support of cash flow to comply with bond covenants are key concerns of lenders and the revenue cycle team.

Other Financial Obligations

While cash flow is affected by payroll, vendor contract payments, interest on debt obligations, capital acquisitions, and possibly the issue of dividends, an organization may have other financial obligations that are not as transparent. Physician contracts, partner distributions, foundation relationships, and community obligations also may make demands on or contribute to cash flow.

In addition to financing from equity and debt instruments, not-for-profit healthcare organizations may have available to them funding from donations directly to patient service funds or other similar foundations. Typically, these donations are solicited to support patient care or long-term projects. For-profit organizations cannot directly benefit from this type of funding.

Financial Statements

At the departmental level, financial transactions are reviewed routinely by department management. For example, the radiology department manager reviews the charges associated with radiology services daily, reconciling the scheduled and unscheduled procedures performed with the recorded transactions. Such review helps to ensure data quality and compliance with policies and procedures. Administrators generally do not review individual transactions. They are more interested in the bottom line summary of the results of transactions. Therefore, summary reports are used to communicate internally with administrators and externally with lending institutions, potential investors, and regulatory agencies. A variety of summaries are useful for analyzing an organization's financial activities. The three key reports are the income statement, the statement of retained earnings, and the balance sheet.

Income Statement

The **income statement** summarizes the organization's revenue and expense transactions during the fiscal year. The statement is also called a *statement of operations* or a *profit-and-loss (P&L) statement*. The income statement reflects the cumulative results of operations between the beginning of the fiscal year and the end of the period for which the statement is being prepared. Income statements can be prepared at any time, but are most commonly prepared monthly, quarterly, and annually.

The arithmetic difference between total revenue and total expenses is **net income.** When total expenses exceed total revenue, net income is a negative number (a **net loss).** When total revenue exceeds total expenses, net income is a positive number (a **net profit**). Net profit increases equity; net loss decreases equity. At the end of the fiscal year, all revenue and expense accounts are closed out and the sum of the balances posted to equity. At the beginning of the new fiscal year, all income statement accounts have a zero balance.

Statement of Retained Earnings

The **statement of retained earnings** (also known as the *statement of changes in fund balance*) expresses changes in retained earnings from the beginning of the balance sheet period to the end. The activity of closing the income statement (revenue and expense) accounts is reflected in the statement of retained earnings. The beginning fund balance for the fiscal year is listed, followed by the cumulative sum of the income statement accounts. If the sum of the balances in the revenue accounts exceeds the sum of the balances in the expense accounts, the change is positive and the ending fund balance is larger than the beginning fund balance. If the sum of the expense account balances exceeds the sum of the revenue account balances, then the change is negative and the ending fund balance is smaller than the beginning fund balance. This statement is, effectively, a snapshot of the impact of organizational activities on the value of the organization. It is also the link between the income statement and the balance sheet.

Balance Sheet

The **balance sheet** is a snapshot of the accounting equation at a point in time. As illustrated earlier in this chapter, every financial transaction affects the accounting equation in some way. Therefore, the balance sheet will change with every transaction. To make the presentation of the balance sheet meaningful, it is typically reviewed on a periodic basis (such as monthly, quarterly, semiannually, and annually) along with an income statement that reflects the same period. Balance sheets are often compared to the prior year's balance sheets at year-end.

The balance sheet lists the major account categories grouped under their accounting equation headings: assets, liabilities, and equity or fund balance. Figure 2.2 shows a set of simple statements, as described earlier in this chapter. The dollar amount shown next to each account category is the total in each category on the ending date listed at the top of the report. Figure 2.3 shows the relationship between the income statement, the statement of retained earnings, and the balance sheet. Note that the financial statements show a number of additional lines not discussed earlier.

All levels of management are included in the annual budget preparation process and should have access to monthly budget reports for their respective departments. Variances in the department budget need to be explained, approved by the department's vice president or the chief financial officer, and submitted to the finance department to assist in determining what changes, if any, need to be made in expected expenses for the remainder of the fiscal year. Budget variances can also affect the financial statements.

Figure 2.2.   Financial statements with the associated income statement and statement of changes in fund balance

Sample Hospital Statement of Revenues and Expenses	12/31/15 (000)
Revenue	
Net patient service revenue	$650
Unrestricted gifts	40
Other	95
Total Revenue	$785
Expenses	
Salaries and wages	$430
Fringe benefits	95
Supplies	175
Total expenses	$700
Income from operations	$ 85
Nonoperating gains	
Unrestricted gifts	$ 15
Excess of revenues over expenses	$100

Sample Hospital Statement of Changes in Unrestricted Fund Balance	2015 (000)
Beginning Balance January 1	$ 900
Excess of Revenues over Expenses	100
Ending Balance December 31	$1,000

Sample Hospital Balance Sheet	12/31/15 (000)
Assets	
Cash	$ 500
Accounts receivable	600
Inventory	400
Building	2,500
Total assets	$4,000
Liabilities	
Accounts payable	600
Mortgage	2,000
Total Liabilities	$2,600
Fund Balance	
Restricted funds	400
Unrestricted funds	1,000
Total Fund Balance	$1,400
Total Liabilities and Fund Balance	$4,000

Source: Davis 2010, 786.

Check Your Understanding 2.2.

1. Review the financial statements shown in figure 2.2. If the net income had been $200,000, what would have been the unrestricted fund balance at the end of the year?

2. Explain the relationship between charges and revenue.

3. How does a group purchasing contract benefit a provider?

Figure 2.3. Relationship between the income statement, statement of changes in fund balance, and the balance sheet

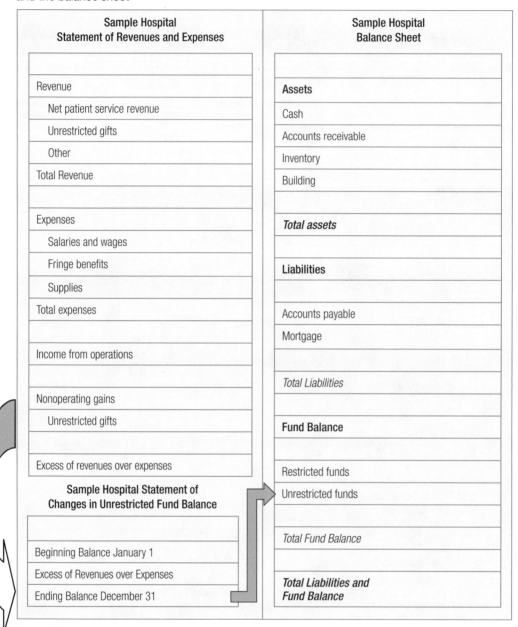

Source: Davis 2010, 787.

The Cost of Providing Services

In a solo practitioner setting, it is relatively simple to identify the costs of providing services. The physician can specifically identify the overhead costs (for example, rent and utilities), salaries, and supplies that are needed as well as the level of income he or she wants to generate from the business. The identification of costs is an essential element in determining whether to participate in a third-party payer's plan. Figure 2.4 shows a simple example of that decision-making process.

Figure 2.4. Sample decision to participate in a managed care contract

Cost of service to be provided:	$200
Charge for service to be provided:	$300
Contracted payer pays 50% of charges: 50% of $300 =	$150

For a solo practitioner, it may not be economically practical to participate in plans for which reimbursement does not cover costs. As mentioned in chapter 1, increasing the volume of patients does not increase the net profit margin if the provider generates a loss on every patient.

For a hospital, the same decision process applies. However, due to the volume, diversity, and complexity of services that are provided by a hospital, the cost analysis and decision process are more difficult. In the current healthcare reimbursement environment, the risk of loss has shifted largely to the providers.

The contract illustrated in figure 2.4 is not advantageous for the hospital because reimbursement is less than the cost of service. However, this contract might be accepted if the payer reimburses for other services more favorably or if this is a portal service that will draw in patients for additional care that is reimbursed more favorably (like a loss leader in a grocery store sale). For example, outpatient laboratory services that barely cover the cost of rendering the care might be a portal or loss-leader for a hospital if the availability of such services encourages patients to have all outpatient services, including high-dollar radiology services, performed at the hospital.

Determining Costs

Before a healthcare organization can reasonably sit down with a payer and negotiate a contract, the organization must answer the following two questions: What are the underlying costs of providing the service(s) under negotiation? How much profit is desired? It is strongly advised that hospitals consider a decision-support system that can run detailed analytics for purposes such as cost accounting, month-end close with reserve calculations, contract and reimbursement management, and contract modeling.

Cost Classification

The term *cost* refers to all of the underlying resources expended to achieve a specific objective. A simple example is the cost of providing a medication to a patient. In addition to the price of the medication itself, the facility also has to pay the pharmacy employees who ordered, stocked, and dispensed the medication as well as the nursing staff who administered the medication. If the medication is dispensed in a paper cup, the facility has to purchase the cup. The facility also has to provide environmental amenities, such as heat and light for the pharmacy and storeroom, and pay other facility employees to dispose of the garbage (such as the medication cup). Yet another expense is the network of individuals and equipment involved in developing and maintaining the physician order-entry system. Suddenly, determining the cost of the medication is not so simple. Understanding how to identify the underlying resources to determine costs begins with three cost classifications: traceability, variability, and controllability.

Traceability

Traceability is the most basic cost classification and has two major categories: direct and indirect costs. **Direct costs** are traceable to a given cost object, whereas **indirect costs** cannot be traced to a given cost object without resorting to some arbitrary method of assignment. A **cost object** is a product (such as the medication in the previous example), process, department, or activity for which the healthcare organization wishes to estimate the cost. When reviewing different cost and budget reports, it is important to understand that the traceability classification can change depending on which cost object is under review. For example, table 2.2 identifies the most common direct and indirect costs when the cost object under consideration is the HIM department. However, if the cost object under consideration is defined as a patient, HIM costs are classified differently (see table 2.3). Most of the direct costs for the HIM department (table 2.2) become indirect costs for the patient (table 2.3), because the department's costs cannot be traced to any specific patient.

Variability

Variability depends on whether the cost is affected by changes in volume. The three most common cost variability categories used are variable, fixed, and mixed. **Variable costs** change as output or volume changes in a constant, proportional manner. An activity that affects or causes costs is called a **cost driver**. **Fixed costs** do not change in response to changes in volume. Some costs are partly variable and partly fixed. To illustrate these costs, consider how coding costs would be classified depending on whether the coders were outsourced contractors or hospital employees. If five full-time employees (FTEs) perform the coding function, salary costs are fixed and do not change as the number of discharges increases or decreases. On the other hand, in an outsourced scenario where the contractual agreement for services is based on a per chart rate, the cost of coding varies in proportion to the volume of discharges. To illustrate mixed cost, assume that the facility has three FTEs who can code 1,000 discharges per month. The cost of coding the first 1,000 discharges is fixed. Any discharges beyond the first 1,000 must be coded by contracted coders, and this cost varies depending on the number of discharges.

Controllability

To facilitate management control, costs also can be categorized as controllable or uncontrollable. **Controllable costs** can be influenced by a department director or manager whereas department managers have little or no effect on **uncontrollable costs**. Effective managers will identify when costs presumed to be uncontrollable can actually be controlled. For example, a department

Table 2.2. Cost object: HIM department

Direct Costs	Indirect Costs
Salaries	Depreciation
Supplies	Housekeeping
Education/training	Utilities
Professional fees	Employee benefits
Software licensing	Maintenance

Table 2.3. Cost object: Patient

Direct Costs from HIM Activities	Indirect Costs from HIM Activities
Supplies	Salaries
	Education/training
	Professional fees
	Software licensing

manager can influence office supply costs, but liability insurance is an uncontrollable cost for department managers because liability insurance is purchased by healthcare facility administrators. Off-site storage may be an uncontrollable cost to a department manager if the storage contract is maintained by central purchasing and the administration dictates the timing of archive storage. However, if the department manager can find cost savings in alternative storage media (historically, microfiche but currently digital scanning of documents) and can make the case to administration, then archiving becomes a controllable cost for the manager.

Cost Allocation

There are four models or methods for the distribution of costs, known as **cost allocation**: the step-down method, the direct method, the double-distribution allocation, and the simultaneous-equations method. The **step-down allocation method** is the method used by CMS when determining the cost of care for Medicare patients. This method involves distributing the costs of nonrevenue, or indirect, departments to other nonrevenue departments and then finally to revenue, or direct, departments. The costs of the nonrevenue departments that serve the most departments, both revenue and nonrevenue, are distributed first. The costs of the nonrevenue department that serve the second-largest number of departments are distributed next.

The attribution of indirect or **overhead costs**, the expenses associated with supporting but not providing patient care services, to revenue-producing service units illustrates the budget concept that all activities must support the mission of the organization. There are four methods of allocation of overhead:

- The direct method of cost allocation distributes the cost of overhead departments solely to the revenue-producing areas. Allocation is based on each revenue-producing area's relative square footage, number of employees, or actual usage of supplies and services. (See table 2.4.)
- The step-down allocation distributes overhead costs once, beginning with the area that provides the least amount of nonrevenue-producing services.
- The double distribution allocates overhead costs twice, which takes into consideration the fact that some overhead departments provide services to each other.
- The simultaneous-equations method distributes overhead costs through multiple iterations, allowing maximum distribution of interdepartmental costs among overhead departments.

The latter three methods of cost allocation listed here assume that overhead cost centers (such as housekeeping) perform services for each other as well as for revenue-producing areas. Therefore, overhead costs are distributed among overhead cost centers as well as revenue-producing areas. Although each of these methods may produce slightly different results, the ultimate goal is to allocate overhead costs appropriately. Appropriate allocation enables the facility to express the full cost of providing services (Davis 2010, 791).

Activity-Based Costing

Activity-based costing (ABC) does not allocate costs but, rather, serves as an economic model that traces the costs or resources necessary for a product or customer. The past two decades have brought substantial changes to healthcare reimbursement. The costs of providing medical services have increased for a variety of reasons, including inflation and medical technology advances. To make informed decisions and remain profitable, a healthcare organization needs accurate cost information. The focus of ABC is to trace costs, especially indirect costs, on the basis of how they are actually consumed and then to control them to improve profitability. This technique identifies the relationship between a significant activity and the resources needed. A major drawback of ABC is that it requires a major investment of resources. Hospitals must redesign their cost

Table 2.4.　Direct allocation versus step-down allocation

	Nonrevenue-Producing Department		Revenue-Producing Department	
	HIM Department	Business Office	Medicine	Laboratory
Direct method:				
Overhead costs before allocation	$360,000	$240,000	$400,000	$250,000
Allocation				
HIM (# discharges processed)	($360,000)		$340,000	$ 20,000
Business office (# labor hours used)		($240,000)	$ 80,000	$160,000
Total overhead after allocation	$　　0	$　　0	$820,000	$430,000
Step-down method:				
Overhead costs before allocation	$360,000	$240,000	$400,000	$250,000
Allocation				
HIM (# discharges processed)	($360,000)	$ 50,000	$300,000	$ 10,000
Business office (# labor hours used)		($290,000)	$ 90,000	$200,000
Total overhead after allocation	$　　0	$　　0	$790,000	$460,000

Source: Davis 2010, 792.

accounting systems, conduct time-consuming interviews, and provide training and education to healthcare personnel regarding ABC principles. Another drawback is that reflecting and analyzing activity-based costs does not necessarily sync with financial accounting practices.

To implement ABC, a healthcare facility must develop two sets of standards: standard cost profiles and standard treatment protocols. A **standard cost profile (SCP)** identifies, analyzes, and defines the activities, including the costs, of departments within the organization to produce a service unit. Developing the SCPs used in ABC requires personnel interviews to determine principal activities to produce a service unit and the amount of time spent on these activities. Most organizations using ABC consider a patient to be the service unit. Just as costs can be categorized as direct and indirect, so can service units. A *direct-service unit* is associated with a specific patient whereas an *indirect-service unit* is provided to another department within a facility. Indirect costs are linked to services through time allocation and other tracing methods. Service units also can be fixed, which means the costs do not change when volume changes. When a facility can provide accurate, detailed cost information related to a specific service, informed decisions can be made. Case-mix and actuarial data can be used to study trends and compare costs by diagnosis, procedure, or attending physician to improve efficiency, reduce waste, and provide a greater understanding of factors affecting cost.

The second component of ABC is **standard treatment protocols (STPs)**. An STP identifies the specific service units necessary to produce a given product. Individual diagnosis-related groups (DRGs) are most often used for inpatient services, and ambulatory payment classifications (APCs) are used for outpatient services. STPs, or clinical pathways, define the optimal care process for a particular diagnosis or surgical procedure.

Healthcare organizations that develop and implement STPs aim to realize two major benefits: the provision of better-quality healthcare and the minimization of costs. Clinical pathways should be developed collaboratively and use a multidisciplinary approach involving clinicians, allied healthcare practitioners, and case managers. As discussed earlier, ABC provides an accurate system to identify and analyze costs. Improved cost data can be merged with clinical data to develop STPs that enhance quality and reduce costs. To improve quality, hospitals should identify best-practice patterns within their own facility and among comparable institutions. Facilities can reduce costs by improving efficiency, reducing redundant interventions, and reducing a patient's length of stay (LOS). Moreover, quality is enhanced through improved patient outcomes and decreased incidence of common complications. Another important benefit of improved cost data and enhanced quality outcomes is improvement in the facility's position in negotiating managed care contracts. Current and future healthcare reforms will continue to stress cost reduction while enhancing the quality of care provided, so STP development and use is expected to increase. In addition to tracing indirect costs, identifying and analyzing SCP and STP data can provide information important for planning, decision-making, ensuring compliance, and follow-up. Implementation of prospective payment systems (PPSs) and associated DRG and APC methodologies have provided hospitals with a logical way to improve strategic decision-making using the customer as the product line or strategic business unit. In healthcare organizations where STPs have been implemented, the quality of coded clinical data has even greater importance in determining a per-case DRG reimbursement amount because it allows for more accurate medical documentation leading to the DRG. Organizations can use aggregate DRG information for strategic planning, budgeting, staffing, **variance analysis** and control, managed care rate setting, assessing and improving patient care quality, outcome measures, and lowering healthcare costs. The quality of coded clinical data will impact healthcare decision making at all levels within the organization.

Although HIM managers are not typically involved in cost-accounting activities, the concepts associated with such activities may prove useful for determining release-of-information fees. The Health Insurance Portability and Accountability Act (HIPAA) requires that fees charged for copies of medical records be based on the cost of providing those copies. While state laws may define maximum rates, these maximums are not generally intended to be set fees but rather a ceiling above which facilities may not charge. The actual cost to provide copies may be significantly lower, particularly in an electronic environment in which copies can be provided at the touch of a button.

HIM Role in Cost Accounting

An HIM manager is not normally directly responsible for cost accounting. However, a basic understanding of cost concepts, including how costs are allocated, is required and will improve the manager's performance in the budget process. Implementation of inpatient and outpatient prospective payment methodologies and the growth of health maintenance organizations (HMOs) and preferred provider organizations (PPOs) have diminished the incidence of cost-based reimbursement, but healthcare organizations still use cost reports and related information, such as a charge description master, to help determine the facilities' costs.

The Charge Description Master

The *charge description master (CDM),* also known as the *chargemaster,* is a database of all the supplies and services provided to patients and the corresponding charges for those items. It enables the facility to capture and record patient charges efficiently as they are incurred. In addition to capturing charges for billing, the CDM can affect budgeting by providing statistics on volume for both individual departments and services. Moreover, charges can be compared to actual costs of providing services to determine the profitability of given services and departments. The CDM is discussed in greater detail in chapter 5.

Medicare Cost Reporting

As described in the following passage from CMS, a **cost report** is an extensive annual report required of facilities that provide services to Medicare patients.

> Medicare-certified institutional providers are required to submit an annual cost report to a Fiscal Intermediary (FI). The cost report contains provider information such as facility characteristics, utilization data, cost and charges by cost center (in total and for Medicare), Medicare settlement data, and financial statement data. CMS maintains the cost report data in the Healthcare Provider Cost Reporting Information System (HCRIS). HCRIS includes subsystems for the Hospital Cost Report (CMS-2552-96), Skilled Nursing Facility Cost Report (CMS-2540-96), Home Health Agency Cost Report (CMS-1728-94), Renal Facility Cost Report (CMS-265-94), and Hospice Cost Report (CMS-1984-99). The data is available in a relational database and consists of every data element included in the HCRIS extract created for CMS by the provider's FI. The data files contain the highest level of Medicare Cost report status; for example, if HCRIS has both an as-submitted report and a final settled report for a specific fiscal year the data files will only contain the final settled report. (CMS 2015)

The Medicare cost reporting data are available on the CMS website and provide valuable benchmarking data for providers and payers alike. To give the reader some sense of the complexity of cost reporting, the summary of hospital cost-report attachments is included in online appendix 2.3.

Medicaid Cost Reporting

Each state's Medicaid program requires that a Medicaid cost report be filed on an annual basis. It is similar to the Medicare cost report and includes a cost-to-charge ratio (CCR) calculation. The CCR from the audited annual Medicaid cost report becomes the hospital's outpatient percent-of-charges reimbursement for the coming fiscal year. The CMS website includes links to each state's Medicaid website for further information about each state-level Medicaid cost-report process.

Determining Charges

The healthcare organization has identified costs for its various services and determined how profitable it needs to be to stay in business. Before negotiating with a payer, it will also want to evaluate the marketplace. What is the competition? How strong is the market share? To what degree does the community support the hospital? What is the regulatory environment in the state? The following discussion is provided to establish a sense of the complexity of the issue of setting charges.

If a provider has one payer that reliably pays 100 percent of charges, then the determination of what to charge is easy—just mark up services to the level of desired profitability or to the extent that the market will bear. However, most providers do not practice in this sort of marketplace. In reality, facilities generally contract with multiple payers reimbursing at different set rates, some of which have nothing to do with charges. However, if a managed care payer agreement uses percent of charges as a reimbursement methodology, there may be language in the rate amendment that limits how much of a CDM increase that payer will allow to be a part of the reimbursement. Medicare, for example, reimburses inpatients at the DRG rate. Although factors such as regional cost of living play a role in the rates that Medicare sets, the charges themselves are largely irrelevant. A commercial payer, on the other hand, might reimburse a per diem rate or a set percentage of charges and base the reimbursement on the lesser of the charges or contracted rate. Therefore, one needs to know whether or not this "lesser of" provision is in the payer rate schedules when determining what CDM rate to set for all payers.

Patients typically care less about the actual price or charge for a service than their out-of-pocket expenses (Clarke 2006). This fact makes public communication about pricing difficult and potentially misleading, creating the need for healthcare providers to measure costs accurately, be cognizant of the marketplace, and ensure that pricing changes maintain the desired net profit

(Clarke 2006). The communication of pricing information to the public is referred to as transparency, which is discussed further in chapters 4 and 7.

Relative Value Unit

The complexity of some settings, such as radiology services and physician practices, makes it impossible to directly calculate a charge per service based on the actual cost to provide that service. In such cases, a **relative value unit (RVU)**—a number derived from the resources used to provide a particular service—can be used both to identify the cost of the service as well as the charge. For example, RVUs enable the physician to distinguish between the resources used to perform a CT scan of the abdomen versus an x-ray of the abdomen. RVUs should take into consideration the fully allocated cost of providing services, as described in the discussion of cost allocation earlier in this chapter.

The calculation of RVUs is dependent on the setting and the desired use of the measure. If there are multiple services offered and the underlying cost of each is known, the RVU is the total cost of each service, divided by the greatest common denominator (GCD) of the services, as shown in table 2.5. In this example, the RVUs of each service can be used to calculate the charges or even to allocate earnings in a practice. RVUs can be as simple or as complex as needed to accurately determine the use of resources to deliver specific services. Medicare uses RVUs for physician reimbursement. The Medicare Part B fee schedule incorporates RVUs for physician work, office expenses, and malpractice expenses. Reimbursement is further adjusted for geographic area.

Hourly Rate

In some settings, prices can be set based on hours. Many therapies can be priced this way. Hourly charges are calculated by taking the total cost for the period plus the desired profit and dividing that sum by the total hours that are anticipated to be charged, as illustrated in figure 2.5.

Table 2.5.   RVU calculation example

	Cost	Greatest Common Denominator (GCD)	RVU
Service 1	$150	5	30
Service 2	$ 75	5	25
Service 3	$ 35	5	7

*Service 1 RVU Cost ($150) / GCD (5) = RVU (30).

Figure 2.5.   Hourly rate calculation example

Total Costs ($750,000) + Profit ($30,000) / Anticipated Hours (5,800) = Hourly Charge Rounded ($135)

Total costs:	$750,000
• Payroll:	$500,000
• Administration:	$100,000
• Supplies:	$130,000
• Overhead:	$ 20,000
Desired profit:	$ 30,000
Total costs plus desired profit:	$780,000
Anticipated service hours:	5,800
Hourly charges (rounded):	$ 135

Surcharge

In some settings, a simple surcharge or overhead rate can be added to the cost of supplies or services to derive the charge. This surcharge can be derived from the relationship between overhead or administrative costs and the overall cost of the service or department. The application of surcharges is a reasonable way to determine the charge for supplies when their price and the fully allocated cost of the department or activity are known. For example, if the total cost of supplies is $1 million and the fully allocated cost of overhead and administrative costs is $250,000, a surcharge of 25 percent (250,000 / 1,000,000) on supplies is required just to cover the cost of handling the supplies (break even). To make a profit, a surcharge in excess of the break-even amount is required.

Cost-to-Charge Ratio

The cost-to-charge ratio (CCR) is developed by taking the total allocated costs for a service, a department, or the entire organization and dividing it by the total charges for the same. For example, if the fully allocated cost of the radiology department is $2 million and the total charges produced by the department in the same period are $2.5 million, the CCR is 2 / 2.5, or 0.80 (80 percent). If a healthcare facility is Medicare certified, its historical CCR can be obtained by reviewing the cost report data on the Medicare website. The Medicaid website publishes the CCR for Medicaid providers. Note that the Medicaid CCR varies from the Medicare CCR because the patient populations of two payers are different, and the differences in the information provided by Medicare versus Medicaid may result in different CCR calculations.

Using the historical CCR to set prices for supplies and services is simple; however, such an approach to pricing may not ultimately give the provider sufficient profit in the current market because reimbursement is not tied to the CCR methodology. Nevertheless, historical CCR is an important benchmark for payers for analytic purposes and may have some relevance to contract negotiations and terms.

Check Your Understanding 2.3.

1. Why is calculating the cost of providing healthcare services so difficult?

2. What is the difference between a variable cost and a fixed cost?

3. List and describe three traditional methods of cost allocation that assume overhead-cost centers perform services for each other as well as for revenue-producing areas.

References

Centers for Medicare and Medicaid Services (CMS). 2015. Cost Reports General Information. https://www.cms .gov/Research-Statistics-Data-and-Systems/Downloadable-Public-Use-Files/Cost-Reports/?redirect= /CostReports/.

Clarke, R. 2006. The real price of transparency. Providers must work to give consumers accurate reading of out-of-pocket costs. *Modern Healthcare.* 36(25):34.

Davis, N. 2010. Financial management. Chapter 25 in *Health Information Management: Concepts, Principles, and Practice,* 3rd ed. Edited by K.M. LaTour and S. Eichenwald Maki. Chicago: AHIMA.

Additional Resources

Cleverley, J. and L. Handlon. 2015. The "lesser of" conundrum: Solving the puzzle through payment terms and the chargemaster. *Strategic Financial Planning.* 10(4):6.

White, S. 2012. *Principles of Finance for Health Information and Informatics Professionals.* Chicago: AHIMA.

Payer Reimbursement

Key Terms

- Abuses
- Ambulatory payment classification (APC)
- Appeal
- Capitation
- Carve out
- Clean claim
- Compliance plan
- Encoder
- Fee-for-service (FFS)
- Fraud
- Grouper
- Home health resource group (HHRG)
- Hospital value-based purchasing (VBP)
- Inpatient prospective payment system (IPPS)
- Inpatient psychiatric facility PPS (IPF PPS)
- Inpatient rehabilitation facility PPS (IRF PPS)
- Office of Inspector General's (OIG's) seven elements
- Outpatient Prospective Payment System (OPPS)
- Positive cash flow
- Relative weight (RW)
- Resource utilization groups, version III (RUG-III)
- Retroactive denials
- Resource-based relative value scale (RBRVS)
- Risk

To negotiate managed care contracts, one must understand the costs of providing services. The reimbursement received must cover costs, and, additionally, the provider must manage the revenue cycle so that cash is received on a timely basis to pay expenses. In chapter 2, we discussed the consideration of cost in terms of the resources used by the practice or facility to provide care. In this chapter, we take that discussion to the next step, which includes cash flow and reimbursement. Although it is assumed that the reader is familiar with the healthcare environment and reimbursement in general, it is useful to review reimbursement methodologies here in the context of provider risk.

Reimbursement Issues

Imagine that you have a great job, a high salary, and you are very good at what you do. You have a mortgage on your home, utilities to pay, and you support a family of four. Based on your stated salary, you should be able to afford the lifestyle you have chosen with no difficulty. But there is a catch—your employer only pays your wages when your work product has been validated. If you make a mistake, you will not be paid until you correct it. If the employer pays you and discovers a mistake later, you have to pay the money back. Now, your mortgage is late and you are looking for a second job to help feed the children. This imagined scenario is analogous to the real-life economics of being a healthcare provider in the United States.

Cash Flow

Cash flow is the cycle of receiving and disbursing cash payments. **Positive cash flow** means that more cash is being received than being disbursed. For a healthcare provider, cash cannot be received until a **clean claim**, a bill devoid of errors and omissions, has been submitted to the payer. Upon payer review, the claim must represent services to a covered individual that are included in the payer-provider contract and have been authorized by the payer, if applicable. Payers will deny payment of claims that do not satisfy this basic criterion or that contain errors or omissions. Therefore, the submission of a clean claim that accurately reflects the services provided is paramount in maintaining positive cash flow. If the payer makes an error and sends more payment than is required by the claim or by the contract, that payer may demand a refund in the future. Payer contracts typically include a look-back period in which claims can be audited and reconciled with the contractual obligation. Data collection for and analysis of claims are discussed in detail in chapters 4 through 7.

Risk

With respect to reimbursement, financial **risk** is the extent to which the provider's revenues might not cover his or her costs. Until the 20th century, the concept of health insurance was relatively unknown. Although various philanthropic and religious organizations have rendered charity care for centuries, the primary payer for healthcare services prior to the 20th century remained the patient. Historically, therefore, the financial relationship of the provider and patient involved just those two parties. The provider's risk in this relationship was that he or she would render services, but the patient would not have the means or desire to pay (reimburse) the provider for those services. As health insurance gained popularity as an employee benefit and with the addition of Medicare and Medicaid to the Social Security program in the United States, the third-party payer has become an increasingly powerful factor in both the reimbursement of healthcare services and the delivery of those services. (Figure 3.1 defines some key health insurance terms.) Thus, with the intervention of the third-party payer, the financial risk evaluation in healthcare reimbursement has grown more complex.

Payers derive revenue from premiums and sponsorship. Therefore, from the payer's perspective, there is the risk that the claims from covered services will exceed the associated revenue stream. Effectively, the payer is betting that the covered lives will remain healthy. As the dollar amount of claims increases, the payer compensates by either reducing covered services or increasing premiums. Other alternatives include changing the reimbursement methodology, as discussed in this chapter.

Centers for Medicare and Medicaid Services Reimbursement Methodologies

There are fundamentally two methods of third-party reimbursement: *fee-for-service (FFS)*, which carries minimal to no risk for payer or provider, and *capitation*, which carries varying degrees of risk, but more for the provider. Both methods have several subcategories. For FFS, these include percent of charges, bundled payments, prospective payment, and hybrids that take from two or more of these concepts to create a hybrid method. These methodologies are incorporated into the contract between the payer and the provider and are driven in large part by the relationship between the two.

Figure 3.1. Insurance terminology

Beneficiary	An individual who is eligible for benefits from a health insurance policy.
Benefit	Healthcare service for which the healthcare insurance company will pay.
Claim	A summary by highest level of coding, whether revenue code on a UB or CPT/HCPCS on a HCFA, of healthcare services and their costs provided by a hospital, physician office, or other healthcare provider; submitted for reimbursement to the healthcare insurance plan by either the insured party or by the provider. If the payer requests to see the charges in more detail; an itemized statement can be provided.
Coinsurance	Method of cost sharing in which the policy or certificate holder pays a pre-established percentage of eligible expenses up until and after the deductible is met, only up until the deductible is met, or only after the deductible is met; the percentage may vary by type or site of service. The application of coinsurance is dependent upon the benefit design.
Coordination of benefits (COB)	A method of integrating benefits payments from all health insurance sources to ensure that they do not exceed 100 percent of a plan member's allowable medical expenses.
Co-payment	Cost-sharing measure in which the policy or certificate holder pays a fixed dollar amount (flat fee) per service, supply, or procedure that is owed to the healthcare facility by the patient. The fixed amount that the policyholder pays may vary by type of service, such as $15 per prescription or $20 per physician visit.
Deductible	The amount of cost, usually annual, the policyholder must incur (and pay) before the insurance plan will assume liability for remaining covered expenses. However, co-pays and co-insurance responsibilities may still be applicable even after the deductible has been met.
Explanation of benefits (EOB)	A statement issued to the insured and the healthcare provider by an insurer to explain the services provided, amounts billed, and payments made by a health plan.
Indemnity or traditional plans	Health insurance coverage provided in the form of cash payments to patients or providers, historically at or close to 100 percent of charges. In the past five to eight years, the industry has seen a significant decline in these type of plans. Instead, indemnity or traditional plans have begun to refer to a less structured and steered plan, meaning no referrals and less pre-certification or authorizations are needed, and a designated primary care physician is not required. Providers are reimbursed at the same rate as managed care products (PPO, HMO, EPO, direct access, etc.). A provider may be paid a higher reimbursement for these plans than the managed care plans, which are more restrictive.
Managed care PPO, EPO, HMO, direct access, etc.	A generic term for reimbursement and delivery systems that integrate the financing and provision of healthcare services by means of entering contractual agreements with selected providers to furnish comprehensive healthcare services and developing explicit criteria for the selection of healthcare providers, formal programs of ongoing quality improvement and utilization review, and significant financial incentives for members to use providers associated with the plan.

Figure 3.1. Insurance terminology (Continued)

Member	The primary insured individual on an insurance policy (enrollee).
Out-of-pocket	Payment made by policyholder or member.
Out-of-pocket expenses	Healthcare costs paid by the insured (for example, deductibles, copayments, and coinsurance) after which the insurer pays a percentage (often 80 or 100 percent) of covered expenses. However, depending upon plan design, the insured may have to pay coinsurance and copayments prior to and after the deductible has been met. Plans today generally have a maximum out-of-pocket limit, which may or may not be set with the deductible as the maximum out–of-pocket expense.
Policies	1. Governing principles that describe how a department or an organization is supposed to handle a specific situation; 2. Binding contracts issued by a healthcare insurance company to an individual or group in which the company promises to pay for healthcare to treat illness or injury; such contracts are also referred to as *health plan agreements* and *evidence of coverage*.
Premium	Amount of money that a policyholder or certificate holder must periodically pay an insurer in return for healthcare coverage.
Provider	Physician, clinic, hospital, nursing home, or other healthcare entity (second party) that delivers healthcare services.
Reimbursement	Compensation or repayment for healthcare services.

Source: AHIMA 2014.

It is essential to understand that the contract between the payer and the insured person (an insurance plan) is entirely different from the contract between the payer and the provider. What follows here is not a discussion of insurance plans, it is a discussion of payer-provider contracts. An individual provider may have multiple contracts or several rate amendments within one contract with the same payer that define specific types of services or site locations within a health system for which the payer will reimburse the provider. Hospitals must charge all patients the same amount regardless of payer (CMS 2016a); therefore, when setting charges, providers must consider the discounts or rates set by various payers. Contract negotiation is a complex process, and providers should ensure that payer terms do not unnecessarily increase the provider's risk.

Fee-for-Service

Fee-for-service (FFS) means that the payer will reimburse the provider an agreed-upon amount for each defined unit of service. The defined unit can be set per diem, per visit, or per unit, or as a percent of charges; it also can be based on diagnosis-related group (DRG). A defined unit of service can be virtually anything the provider does for the patient, such as a laboratory test, radiology examination, inpatient day of care, or physical therapy. Every service that a provider offers should be included in the contract with the payer. If the payer does not reimburse for a particular service, then that should be spelled out in the contract.

The risk for the payer in an FFS contract is largely that services reimbursed at agreed-upon amounts will exceed the associated revenue stream from premiums. This excess can happen in at least two ways: the agreed-upon payment amount is too high or the number of covered individuals seeking those services exceeds predicted rates, meaning the severity of illness of covered individuals is greater than predicted. The payer can ameliorate the risk of high payment rates by being very specific in its provider contract. The latter two risks can be controlled by capping the dollar amount or frequency of usage by covered individuals. For example, the payer may limit coverage of physical therapies to a set number of visits per covered event or contract year. These limits are determined by the payer when the patient is fully insured or by the employer when the patient is self-insured. If an employer group is self-insured, that group can set limits (based on guidance from the payer) to limit or increase the employer's out-of-pocket financial exposure, just as the payer does with fully insured plan options.

The risk to the provider in an FFS contract is, therefore, not just that the cost of providing care will exceed the reimbursement but also that the patient's coverage for those services has exceeded the aforementioned limits. The importance of not only identifying insurance coverage for an incoming patient but also verifying the extent to which the current episode of care will be reimbursed is a critical patient access function, as discussed in chapter 4.

Fee-for-service describes the vast preponderance of contracts between payers and providers. Within the FFS methodology are numerous ways of calculating the reimbursement amount, including fee schedules, per diem or per admission amounts (which are also called case rates or DRG-based rates), and prospective payment. For example, the payer may reimburse at a per diem rate for inpatient stays, use a fee schedule for outpatient services, and prospective payment for ambulatory surgery. In addition, the payer may agree to **carve out** (pay separately for) certain supplies and high-cost services. For example, an inpatient stay would be paid at a per diem rate, but high-cost drugs administered during the stay would be reimbursed separately. Further, FFS payments may be increased or decreased by performance-based criteria, such as patient outcomes. These types of pay-for-performance methodologies will be covered in more detail later in this chapter. Among the FFS reimbursement methodologies is Medicare's prospective payment system (PPS), which is summarized in table 1.4.

Prospective Payment System

Prospective payment is the term used to indicate that the payment for a particular type of service has been decided prior to the service being provided to the patient. Most often it is called the prospective payment system (PPS). PPS is the primary reimbursement method used for reimbursement of services provided to Medicare beneficiaries, although other payers also use PPS models, or a variation of them, as a method of payment. For example, when a managed care payer uses this methodology, they may incorporate a percentage of the provider's Medicare base rate and then follow Medicare's weight-adjustment methodology. Such payers often attach the calculated DRG as a fee schedule to the contract rather than expect the weights to be calculated with each claim submission, as discussed below.

The first PPS, called DRGs, was implemented in 1983. The Balanced Budget Act (BBA) of 1997 brought about additional PPS methods for other Medicare services reimbursement. These PPS methods are determined by a study of prior services and the charges associated with each particular type of service. When the system is set, all future payments for each service can be determined prior to patient care and adjusted by the Centers for Medicare and Medicaid Services (CMS) for Medicare payment, as needed, to control spending. The adjustments and changes in the system are published annually in the *Federal Register* prior to implementation, first as a proposed rule and then, after a comment period, as a final rule. For each PPS discussed, accurate coding and appropriate documentation of patient care remain critically important. To determine appropriate payment, documentation is required to support the coding that is performed. The following section is a high-level introduction to the various PPSs. The emphasis on inpatient methodology in this text mirrors the greater influence that inpatient services, and the HIM staff coding for inpatient billing, have on the revenue cycle. Most often, greater revenue is available per inpatient account versus per outpatient account. For detailed coverage, see Casto's and Forrestal's *Principles of Healthcare Reimbursement*, which is listed under resources at the end of this chapter.

Diagnosis-Related Groups

DRGs are a component of the **inpatient prospective payment system (IPPS)** developed for reimbursement of Medicare hospital inpatient claims. A DRG is determined by assignment of the appropriate International Classification of Diseases, Tenth Revision, Clinical Modification (ICD-10-CM) and International Classification of Diseases, Tenth Revision, Procedure Coding System (ICD-10-PCS) codes for the principal diagnosis, any surgical procedures, complications, comorbidities as required by coding guidelines, and patient age. DRGs are organized into three segments: pregrouping, major diagnostic categories (MDCs), and other. Pregrouping DRGs include transplants, tracheostomies, and ventilator support. The other section includes major surgical procedures that are not related to the principal diagnosis. The rest of the DRGs are grouped in the appropriate diagnosis-related MDCs, which are further partitioned by medical and surgical groups. Table 3.1 includes a list of diagnoses that are related by body system (for example, a myocardial infarction would be assigned to the cardiovascular MDC). The assignment of a DRG is accomplished through the use of a software program called a **grouper**, which applies a series of logical steps, illustrated in figure 3.2, to assign prospective payment groups on the basis of clinical codes (AHIMA 2014). A patient can be assigned to only one DRG for a specific inpatient visit. CMS assigns each DRG a **relative weight (RW)**, which reflects the relative resource consumption associated with a payment classification or group (AHIMA 2014). RW is used to determine the hospital's reimbursement for that particular DRG. The RW is also used to calculate a case-mix index (CMI).

Table 3.1. DRG language

Major Diagnostic Category (MDC)	List of diagnoses that are related, predominantly by body system
Partition	The two subcategories of an MDC: surgical and medical.
Comorbidity/complication (CC)	A designation assigned to a secondary diagnosis that reflects the additional resources needed to treat a patient with that condition. This designation is not absolute. Some diagnoses are CCs whenever they appear, such as F05, Delirium due to known physiological condition; others are CCs only in combination with specific principal diagnoses.
Major comorbidity/complication (MCC)	Similar to CCs, a designation assigned to a limited number of secondary diagnoses that reflect significant additional resources needed to treat a patient with that condition. For example, J18.9, Pneumonia, unspecified organism, is currently an MCC that applies to all principal diagnoses. As with CCs, MCCs do not apply in combination with all principal diagnoses.

Figure 3.2. Basic DRG grouper logic

1. Do the procedure codes reflect a pre-MDC procedure? If yes, assign DRG to the appropriate code in the list. If no, go on to step 2.
2. Identify the MDC under which the diagnosis is listed.
3. Within the MDC, identify whether there is a surgical procedure. If yes, refer to the surgical partition within the MDC. If no, refer to the medical partition within the MDC.
4. Within the partition, match the principal diagnosis to the appropriate subcategory. Based on the secondary diagnoses, the DRG selection depends on whether there is a comorbidity/complication (CC) or a major comorbidity/complication (MCC).
5. Some special rules apply, such as when a case is ungroupable or if there is a major surgical procedure that is unrelated to the principal diagnosis. In both cases, there is a special DRG to capture these few situations.

In the HIM department, an encoder—software designed to look up codes based on the diagnosis or procedure description—is used to help the coding staff assign the correct ICD-10-CM and ICD-10-PCS codes. Some encoders are composed of a series of menus that prompt the user to select descriptors until a matching code results. Other encoders are used primarily as electronic code books. All encoders contain some level of support for the user in the form of reference material, which may include a medical dictionary, an anatomy and physiology reference, a pharmaceutical reference, and coding resources such as Coding Clinic and CPT Assistant—the major industry guides to correct coding.

Version 24 of the Medicare DRG data set and grouper was the last version prior to the CMS expansion and adjustment of DRGs to refine reimbursement for severity of illness. The version 24 grouper is sometimes called the "classic" version for this reason. Beginning with version 25, Medicare moved to a severity-adjusted model called Medicare severity diagnosis-related groups (MS-DRGs). CMS evaluates Medicare claims data to ensure that the groupings stay current with changes in the coding classification as well as changes in clinical practice. Thus, the implementation of ICD-10-CM/PCS in October 2015 required an overhaul of the MS-DRG grouper for version 33.

Resource-Based Relative Value Scale

The **resource-based relative value scale (RBRVS)** is used for physician reimbursement for services covered by Medicare Part B. It results in the annually published Medicare Part B fee schedule, which can be downloaded by state from the CMS website. The fee schedule includes split billing to show reimbursement rates for the physician versus rates for the facility in which an outpatient service or procedure was rendered. The physician uses the CMS-1500 form, shown in figure 3.3, or its electronic equivalent (which is called 837p) to submit claims to the Medicare carrier for reimbursement. The Medicare carrier, or Medicare administrative contractor (MAC), processes outpatient claims for the federal government. Reimbursement is based on the Current Procedural Terminology/Healthcare Common Procedure Coding System (CPT/HCPCS) procedure codes, and ICD-10-CM diagnosis codes support the medical necessity of the procedure(s).

Ambulatory Payment Classification

An **ambulatory payment classification (APC)** is a component of the hospital **outpatient prospective payment system (OPPS)** and pertains to hospital outpatient services, certain Medicare Part B services furnished to hospital inpatients who have no Part A coverage, and partial hospitalization services furnished by community mental health centers (CMS 2015a). APCs specifically cover the reimbursement for outpatient procedures defined as same-day surgery (SDS), same-day medical (SDM), and minor procedures (MP). This methodology can be used as part of the outpatient fee schedules when negotiating with payers. As with Medicare, managed care payers reimburse APCs on a per case basis, although some implantable procedures or other high-dollar services may be carved out and reimbursed in addition to the per case rate. APCs are based on HCPCS, which has the following two levels:

- Level I: CPT codes
- Level II: HCPCS codes

APCs reflect the procedures performed. There may be more than one APC per encounter. To determine payment, an APC refers to the status indicator assigned to the CPT/HCPCS code(s). Some procedures (status code T) result in reduced payment when they are performed at the same time as other procedures, or when other procedures are bundled. Table 3.2 shows the status indicators and their impact on reimbursement. Managed care payers that use APCs to determine reimbursement may use a variety of calculations, such as paying their full rate for all APCs on the

Figure 3.3.   A sample physician practice bill on a CMS-1500 form

HEALTH INSURANCE CLAIM FORM

APPROVED BY NATIONAL UNIFORM CLAIM COMMITTEE (NUCC) 02/12

PICA

1. MEDICARE   MEDICAID   TRICARE   CHAMPVA   GROUP HEALTH PLAN   FECA BLK LUNG   OTHER   1a. INSURED'S I.D. NUMBER (For Program in Item 1)
(Medicare#) (Medicaid#) (ID#/DoD#) (Member ID#) (ID#) (ID#) (ID#)

2. PATIENT'S NAME (Last Name, First Name, Middle Initial)
3. PATIENT'S BIRTH DATE   SEX
4. INSURED'S NAME (Last Name, First Name, Middle Initial)

5. PATIENT'S ADDRESS (No., Street)
6. PATIENT RELATIONSHIP TO INSURED   Self Spouse Child Other
7. INSURED'S ADDRESS (No., Street)

CITY   STATE
8. RESERVED FOR NUCC USE
CITY   STATE

ZIP CODE   TELEPHONE (Include Area Code)
ZIP CODE   TELEPHONE (Include Area Code)

9. OTHER INSURED'S NAME (Last Name, First Name, Middle Initial)
10. IS PATIENT'S CONDITION RELATED TO:
11. INSURED'S POLICY GROUP OR FECA NUMBER

a. OTHER INSURED'S POLICY OR GROUP NUMBER
a. EMPLOYMENT? (Current or Previous) YES NO
a. INSURED'S DATE OF BIRTH   SEX

b. RESERVED FOR NUCC USE
b. AUTO ACCIDENT? YES NO   PLACE (State)
b. OTHER CLAIM ID (Designated by NUCC)

c. RESERVED FOR NUCC USE
c. OTHER ACCIDENT? YES NO
c. INSURANCE PLAN NAME OR PROGRAM NAME

d. INSURANCE PLAN NAME OR PROGRAM NAME
10d. CLAIM CODES (Designated by NUCC)
d. IS THERE ANOTHER HEALTH BENEFIT PLAN? YES NO   If yes, complete items 9, 9a, and 9d.

READ BACK OF FORM BEFORE COMPLETING & SIGNING THIS FORM.
12. PATIENT'S OR AUTHORIZED PERSON'S SIGNATURE I authorize the release of any medical or other information necessary to process this claim. I also request payment of government benefits either to myself or to the party who accepts assignment below.
SIGNED   DATE
13. INSURED'S OR AUTHORIZED PERSON'S SIGNATURE I authorize payment of medical benefits to the undersigned physician or supplier for services described below.
SIGNED

14. DATE OF CURRENT ILLNESS, INJURY, or PREGNANCY (LMP)   QUAL.
15. OTHER DATE   QUAL.
16. DATES PATIENT UNABLE TO WORK IN CURRENT OCCUPATION   FROM   TO

17. NAME OF REFERRING PROVIDER OR OTHER SOURCE
17a.
17b. NPI
18. HOSPITALIZATION DATES RELATED TO CURRENT SERVICES   FROM   TO

19. ADDITIONAL CLAIM INFORMATION (Designated by NUCC)
20. OUTSIDE LAB? YES NO $ CHARGES

21. DIAGNOSIS OR NATURE OF ILLNESS OR INJURY Relate A-L to service line below (24E)   ICD Ind.
A.   B.   C.   D.
E.   F.   G.   H.
I.   J.   K.   L.
22. RESUBMISSION CODE   ORIGINAL REF. NO.
23. PRIOR AUTHORIZATION NUMBER

24. A. DATE(S) OF SERVICE From To   B. PLACE OF SERVICE   C. EMG   D. PROCEDURES, SERVICES, OR SUPPLIES (Explain Unusual Circumstances) CPT/HCPCS MODIFIER   E. DIAGNOSIS POINTER   F. $ CHARGES   G. DAYS OR UNITS   H. EPSDT Family Plan   I. ID. QUAL.   J. RENDERING PROVIDER ID. #

1   NPI
2   NPI
3   NPI
4   NPI
5   NPI
6   NPI

25. FEDERAL TAX I.D. NUMBER   SSN EIN
26. PATIENT'S ACCOUNT NO.
27. ACCEPT ASSIGNMENT? (For govt. claims, see back) YES NO
28. TOTAL CHARGE $
29. AMOUNT PAID $
30. Rsvd for NUCC Use

31. SIGNATURE OF PHYSICIAN OR SUPPLIER INCLUDING DEGREES OR CREDENTIALS (I certify that the statements on the reverse apply to this bill and are made a part thereof.)
SIGNED   DATE
32. SERVICE FACILITY LOCATION INFORMATION
a. b.
33. BILLING PROVIDER INFO & PH #
a. b.

NUCC Instruction Manual available at: www.nucc.org   PLEASE PRINT OR TYPE   APPROVED OMB-0938-1197 FORM 1500 (02-12)

CARRIER — PATIENT AND INSURED INFORMATION — PHYSICIAN OR SUPPLIER INFORMATION

claim or using a tiered reimbursement method that pays 100 percent of the primary procedure payment rate, 50 percent of the secondary payment rate, and either 25 percent or 0 percent of the payment rate for any procedure thereafter.

Resource Utilization Groups, Version III

Resource utilization groups, version III (RUG-III) is the per diem reimbursement method used for Medicare patients in skilled nursing facilities; it is based on the Minimum Data Set (MDS 3.0),

Table 3.2. OPPS payment status indicators and description of payment under OPPS

Status Indicator	Description of Payment under OPPS
SI A	Services paid under some other method (such as a fee schedule): • Ambulance services • Clinical diagnostic laboratory services • Nonimplantable prosthetic and orthotic devices • EPO for ESRD patients • Physical, occupational, and speech therapy • Routine dialysis services for ESRD patients provided in a certified dialysis unit of a hospital • Diagnostic mammography • Screening mammography
SI B	Codes that are not recognized by OPPS when submitted on an outpatient hospital Part B bill type
SI C	Inpatient procedures
SI D	Discontinued codes
SI E	Items, codes, and services not covered by Medicare
SI F	Corneal tissue acquisition; certain CRNA services and Hepatitis B vaccines
SI G	Pass-through drugs and biologicals
SI H	Pass-through device categories
SI K	Non-pass-through drugs, nonimplantable biologicals, and therapeutic
SI L	Influenza vaccine; Pneumococcal pneumonia vaccine
SI M	Items and services not billable to the fiscal intermediary/MAC
SI N	Items and services packaged into APC rates
SI P	Partial hospitalization
SI Q	Packaged services subject to separate payment under OPPS payment criteria
SI Q1	STVX-Packaged codes
SI Q2	T-Packaged codes
SI Q3	Codes that may be paid through a composite APC
SI R	Blood and blood products
SI S	Significant procedure, not discounted when multiple
SI T	Significant procedure, multiple reduction applies
SI U	Brachytherapy services
SI V	Clinic or emergency department visit
SI Y	Nonimplantable durable medical equipment
SI X	Ancillary services

which is part of the facility's required patient documentation in the resident assessment instrument. MDS 3.0 was implemented on October 1, 2009. The MDS 3.0 information is collected and submitted electronically by the provider via the Resident Assessment Validation and Entry (RAVEN) software. "RAVEN imports and exports data in standard MDS record format; maintains facility, resident, and employee information; enforces data integrity via rigorous edit checks; and provides comprehensive on-line help. It includes a data dictionary and a RUG calculator" (Hazelwood and Venable 2014, 274). CMS also uses the Data Assessment and Verification (DAVE) program to determine accuracy of the MDS and ensure that it does not pay facilities more than they have earned. The importance of documentation timeliness and accuracy must be stressed in this and all PPS methods. RUG-III is not a case-based (one-payment) methodology. Rather, it is a periodic assessment of the patient's status that results in corresponding payments to the provider. Hence, accurate calculation is needed at every submission.

Home Health Resource Groups

Home health resource groups (HHRGs) comprise the PPS for Medicare home health patient care reimbursement. The system is composed of 80 HHRGs. The HHRG is determined by Outcomes and Assessment Information Set (OASIS) data. Like skilled nursing facilities, home health agencies need to use a designated system for submitting patient information. Their system, called the Home Assessment Validation and Entry (HAVEN), is used to capture and submit OASIS data electronically within seven days of the start of care and periodically thereafter. While the OASIS data contain the majority of information about patient status, the ICD-10-CM codes are critical to ensuring that OASIS data accurately convey the patient's diagnostic status.

Inpatient Psychiatric Facility PPS

The **inpatient psychiatric facility PPS (IPF PPS)** is a per diem PPS based on 15 DRGs and a variety of adjustment factors, including age and comorbidity. Because the highest cost incurred by the IPF is at the beginning of the patient admission, the per diem reimbursement rate varies, with the highest rate on the first day of admission, decreasing rates through the eighth day, and no adjustment thereafter. Patient-level adjustments to payments are made for the patient's age as well as certain MS-DRGs and comorbidities, a fact that once again points to the need for accurate coding. Facilities may also be eligible for outlier payments when costs for a specific case exceed specified limits. Additional information on the IPF PPS can be found on the CMS website (CMS 2015b).

Inpatient Rehabilitation Facility PPS

The **inpatient rehabilitation facility PPS (IRF PPS)** uses the patient assessment instrument (PAI) to assign patients in inpatient rehabilitation facilities to 1 of 97 case-mix groups according to their clinical healthcare financial environment situation and resource requirements. The PAI, which must be completed by the third day after admission, can be collected and submitted electronically using the Inpatient Rehabilitation Validation and Entry (IRVEN) system made available free of charge by CMS. Like HAVEN and RAVEN, IRVEN benefits both the inpatient rehabilitation facility and CMS. Diagnosis coding for IRF PPS can be somewhat confusing because the codes normally assigned per UB-04 guidelines do not necessarily match those required for PAI data. The principal diagnosis listed on the UB-04 (837i) would be "encounter for rehabilitation," whereas the PAI is looking specifically for the codes for the functional impairment and the etiology of the impairment. A *Journal of AHIMA* article published in 2007 covers the challenges of IRF PPS (Trela 2007). Additional and current information on the IRF PPS are on the CMS website (CMS 2013).

Non-Medicare Groupers

Because Medicare is a federal benefit for the elderly and disabled population, the PPS (DRGs) designed for Medicare is not sufficient for use with all patients in the healthcare system. Those systems used to analyze groups of patients that are not eligible for Medicare (for example, systems used for reimbursement for Medicaid recipients) are called *non-Medicare groupers*. (See table 3.3.) As mentioned previously, these systems are modified variations of the Medicare DRG system. Most of the modified systems are designed by 3M. For example, the State of New York contracted with 3M to design the all-patient DRG (AP-DRG). This is notable because commercial payers may negotiate contracts that require the use of a grouper that is not the current grouper

Table 3.3. Select Non-Medicare groupers

Grouper	Acronym	Description
All-patient diagnosis-related group (DRG)	AP-DRG	Modified version of DRG system used by the State of New York
Refined-DRG	R-DRG	Modified version of the DRG system that considered the CC in addition to the principal diagnosis and procedures for a patient. The design included four CC-complexity levels based on the number and intensity of CCs: non-CC, moderate-CC, major-CC, and catastrophic-CC
All-patient refined DRG	APR-DRG	AP-DRGs modified for severity of illness and risk of mortality
Severity-DRGs	SDRG	Does not include DRGs for pediatrics, pregnancy, and newborns

being used by Medicare. It is also worth noting that not all payers are required to implement ICD-10-CM/PCS. For example, workers' compensation and auto-medical payers may still be using ICD-9-CM and therefore cannot use the current Medicare grouper.

Capitation

A **capitation** contract reimburses the provider a set amount per covered individual per month; this is referred to as the *per member per month (PMPM) rate*. The provider is then responsible for a specific set of services to be rendered to that individual. Some additional reimbursement may be obtained for costly or lengthy procedures. An underlying assumption is that the payer-patient contract requires the up-front selection and identification of a specific provider by the patient and financial incentives to encourage the patient to seek care from that provider. For example, the patient chooses a primary care physician (PCP) and pays little or no out-of-pocket costs for care from that PCP. However, the patient would be responsible for reimbursement for care received from a different PCP.

The risk of financial loss in a capitation arrangement rests with the provider. For example, specialists who provide services on referral will not be reimbursed without an appropriate referral. The payer's financial obligation is, for the most part, discharged with the period-fixed payments to the provider. On the provider's side, the fixed payments provide a predictable revenue stream. However, since the revenue is not entirely linked to services, the provider is at financial risk if a higher-than-predicted percentage of the panel (the patients assigned to that provider) uses the provider's services. Table 3.4 illustrates the financial risk for the provider that is inherent in capitation.

Pay-for-Performance and Potential Reduction in Reimbursement Risks (Quality/Patient Safety Programs)

While the provider assumes the full financial risk in a capitation agreement with a payer, P4P agreements offer a modified-risk arrangement for the provider. At this time, P4P is not a reimbursement methodology and generally does not stand alone as the payer's only form of payment for services a provider renders. As previously mentioned, in addition to FFS reimbursement, providers can be paid additional money for achieving quality patient care while reducing costs. Medicare and the managed care companies' accountable care organization (ACO) models are examples of this shared-savings concept. An ACO consists of a group of providers—physicians, hospitals, and nonacute care facilities—that combine to provide high-quality coordinated care across settings. The ACO itself may be a single entity that employs or owns the various providers, or it may be a contractual entity in which some or all of the providers are otherwise

Table 3.4. Provider risk in capitation: Costs exceeding capitation payments

Number of Patients	Visits per Month	Cost to Provide Service	Total Cost
890	0	$ 0	$ 0
100	1	$20	$2,000
10	Hospitalized	$60	$ 600
Total cost of services to the 1,000-patient panel			$2,600
Monthly capitation payment			$2,000 ($2/patient)
Cost in excess of payment in this month			$ 600

independent of the ACO. Medicaid ACOs, which are similar to Medicare ACOs, are being rolled out state by state.

The purpose of ACOs and other versions of P4P programs is to establish quality patient care while reducing healthcare costs. One typical area of focus is emergency department (ED) visits. The P4P goal is for physicians to keep their patients out of the ED and, when possible, treat patients in a more appropriate—and less costly—healthcare environment, such as an urgent care center or the physician's office. Generally, the shift from care in the ED to care in other settings lowers the provider's volume of services and reduces payments from the payer. This shift could therefore be a potential financial risk for the provider; however, in a P4P program, the payer shares a predetermined percentage of its savings from reduced healthcare costs with the provider, which thereby helps lower the provider's financial risk.

Patient-Centered Medical Homes

The desire to reduce healthcare costs while maintaining the highest quality care has also resulted in the creation of patient-centered medical homes (PCMHs). A PCMH's focus is usually on primary care, but specialist and multispecialty PCMHs also exist. The PCMH's role is to manage patient care from the PCP's perspective and thereby prevent duplicate ancillary services such as blood work or radiology services. PCMHs are most successful at managing patients at higher risk whose care is costlier than the care of the average healthier patient, who is served better within the ACO model. Successful PCMHs are usually certified by the National Committee for Quality Assurance (NCQA). NCQA certification signifies to a payer that the provider has an established high-quality clinical program with the ability to reduce healthcare costs.

Value-Based Purchasing

The **hospital value-based purchasing (VBP)** program adjusts Medicare's payments to reward hospitals that achieve specified parameters for quality of care. The program reduces participating hospitals' Medicare payments by a specified percentage. It then uses estimated total amounts of the reduced payment to fund the VBP payments to hospitals based on each hospital's individual performance against the quality measures specified by the program.

The deduction is taken off the hospital's base operating DRG payment amount. This program began in 2013 with a 1.0 percent reduction to participating hospitals' base rates. The reduction increases by 0.25 percent per year until 2017, when it will stabilize at a 2.0 percent annual reduction for 2017 and onward. The second payment adjustment is applied at the time of payment on a claim-by-claim basis based on the hospital's total performance score (TPS), which is based on the VBP program's overall measures. Once the TPS factor is calculated, it is multiplied by the base operating DRG payment amount on a claim-by-claim basis. The specific quality measures that contribute to the TPS can be reviewed on Medicare's website (42 CFR 412.160).

Meaningful Use

As part of the American Recovery and Reinvestment Act of 2009, the Health Information Technology for Economical and Clinical Health (HITECH) Act has provided financial incentives, called meaningful use payments, to physicians and hospitals for implementing electronic medical record or electronic health record (EMR/EHR) systems. The rationale for implementing EMR/EHR systems is to appropriately share medical data, which helps achieve the interoperability that ACO and PCMH models need to succeed. In order to receive meaningful use payments and to qualify for participation in the next phase of the incentive program, providers must meet specific criteria and are subject to audits that take place at the end of each year. Phases 1 and 2 are complete, and phase 3 will be finalized by the end of 2016. CMS recently announced that the meaningful use program will transition from a focus on technology implementation to a focus on improving the quality of patient care through the technology (Butler 2016).

Delivery System Reform Incentive Payment

The delivery system reform incentive payment (DSRIP) is a type of Medicaid "patient quality of care" program, and participation in DSRIP is one of the criteria for states to receive federal funding to expand Medicaid. Before the introduction of DSRIP, disproportionate share hospital (DSH) dollars were allocated to hospitals within each state based solely on financial need, which was assessed using the number of Medicaid and charity care recipients served in the state. When DSRIP was created, it replaced the existing DSH program. The payments are now redistributed based solely on the quality of the approved program in which the hospital selects to participate. Approval to participate in a program is based on state-published criteria. (Criteria can vary by state.) For example, in 2014 New Jersey's DSRIP program allowed all hospitals to begin applying for acceptance. As with meaningful use, hospitals must meet all of the current year's criteria to continue in the program the next year. DSRIP-type funding is unique and at the forefront of healthcare reform because hospitals that previously did not qualify for DSH funds can now qualify for DSRIP funds based on the quality of their program. However, the reverse is also true; hospitals that automatically qualified for DSH dollars may no longer qualify if they do not meet the quality criteria of the DSRIP program.

To continue to qualify for federal and state funds through programs like DSRIP, large health systems have had to create ACO-type programs designed to offer quality care and reduce healthcare expenses for patients with, for example, asthma, diabetes, heart disease, or behavioral health diagnoses. Hospitals are expected to identify patients eligible for these programs by using data in their systems and must ask these patients to agree to be treated in their DSRIP-funded program. The DSRIP program also involves outreach to organizations such as homeless shelters and senior citizen groups within the hospital's community. Hospitals put forth a significant amount of time and effort in these types of programs to avoid a negative financial impact on the hospital.

Other Opportunities for Revenue Based on P4P

Medicare and Medicaid also financially reward PCPs who improve the quality of care by documenting the patient's responses to certain questions, such as tobacco and alcohol use, asked during the physician's evaluation of specific body systems, such as the cardiovascular, pulmonary, and endocrine systems. The patient-response data help the physician ascertain at each visit the patient's risk of comorbidities related to high-dollar diagnoses such as heart and lung diseases and diabetes.

Another quality and patient-safety program having a financial impact on providers is the hospital-acquired conditions (HAC) program, which can result in reduced or no reimbursement depending upon the payer. (See chapter 6 for further discussion of the HAC program.) It is important to keep in mind that P4P or quality and patient-safety programs can be found within commercial-payer agreements, too. The concept is not exclusive to Medicare and Medicaid and therefore needs to be taken into account during the contract negotiations modeling process discussed later in this chapter.

Medicare policy changes, which occur routinely, are a potential risk to the P4P programs. Medicare is in the process of raising the bar for collaboration between hospitals and physicians to reduce readmission rates by penalizing hospitals for readmissions that occur within 30 days. Hospitals need to work very closely with physicians to ensure that patients do not go home too quickly, and, more importantly, both the hospital and the attending physician must have a follow-up discharge plan to help the patient once he or she is back at home. This discharge plan is expected to include follow-up doctor's appointments and medication-compliance checks. This process is not easy for a hospital to implement because its usual role in patient care ends at the time of discharge. Since the financial impact of readmission penalties can be significant to the hospital, hospital case-management and nursing administration now think very differently about discharge planning, including, but not limited to, the use of patient care coordinators (PCCs) who follow up with the patient and the patient's PCP to try to ensure that the patient is complying with the discharge plan. For example, a PCC might follow up with a recently discharged patient to verify that the patient has made a follow-up appointment with their PCP, obtained their prescribed medication, and enacted any necessary behavior modifications. A patient's failure to comply with the discharge plan may result in a worsening of his or her condition and a subsequent readmission.

Another type of P4P to consider is the higher risk concept of bundled payments. Under this model, reimbursement for all providers within the continuum of care for a specific patient's care, such as for breast cancer or knee replacement surgery, would be bundled into one payment that all providers have to share. Quality care in the right setting at the minimum costs is the goal of this, or any other, payer and provider collaboration. All the patient's care providers, whether in-home, at the hospital outpatient department, or in a freestanding outpatient center, must work together on the patient's care plan to ensure that no services, including outpatient tests, are unnecessarily duplicated. Care providers must also ensure that the patient is not using services such as physical therapy for too long; thus, a PCC might be charged with making sure that the patient does the prescribed at-home exercises. The complexity of even these simple examples illustrates the need for hospitals and physicians to collaborate in caring for the patient mindfully as he or she moves between settings.

Interoperability, the ability of different information systems and software applications to communicate and exchange data (AHIMA 2014, 82), is the largest challenge to PCMH programs, ACOs, and other P4P concepts that CMS or the managed care payers roll out to providers. For example, the hospital must be able to notify the PCP of an admission and collaborate with that physician, as needed, regarding the patient's care. This collaborative communication is most easily accomplished through a notification system that links the hospital's systems with the PCP's. However, such interoperability does not necessarily exist. When it does not, communications typically occur in a series of phone calls, e-mails, or faxes that are not automatically captured in the electronic records and require manual tracking. Providers' ability to share the necessary medical records requires full integration of the computer systems belonging to the PCP, specialists, hospitals, freestanding facilities (surgery centers, urgent care, radiology), laboratories, and other healthcare providers. Finally, the ability to communicate quickly and efficiently with the payers for notification of admissions, continuing care authorizations, and submission of supporting documentation should not be ignored. Ultimately, all of the aforementioned parties may be linked through a health information exchange (HIE), in which the various entities will have to connect with only the HIE rather than each other individually, similar to the way that providers connect with payers through a clearinghouse. Until then, manual workarounds will continue to be employed.

Compliance

Any lack of compliance has the potential to affect a provider's financial situation, at least through the imposition of fines and other financial penalties; however, there are a number of compliance issues that are directly related to the revenue cycle. Providers must maintain compliance with federal and state regulations in all negotiations with payers or other providers. Important federal regulations that must be considered include the following:

- The Sherman Anti-Trust Act, which prohibits contracts that result in restraint of trade
- The Clayton Act, which strengthens the Sherman Anti-Trust Act and established the Federal Trade Commission
- The False Claims Act, which makes defrauding governmental programs a federal crime
- The Operation Restore Trust, which establishes a federal-state partnership to combat healthcare fraud, waste, and abuse
- The criminal disclosure provision of the Social Security Act, which imposes civil and criminal penalties for fraudulent activities
- Stark II Law, which prohibits "kickbacks" (compensation for referrals)
- The Health Insurance Portability and Accountability Act (HIPAA), which addresses monitoring of federal exclusion lists and conflicts of interest
- The Emergency Medical Treatment and Active Labor Act (EMTALA), which prohibits facilities from "dumping" patients in potentially emergent or urgent situations (such as women in active labor or patients possibly experiencing cardiac arrest) due to inability to pay, and which requires that insurance plans reimburse the facility for the services rendered even if the "emergency" turns out to be a nonurgent problem (such as indigestion instead of a heart attack)

Both HIM and patient financial services (PFS) professionals must conform to all legal and regulatory aspects of their job functions, as evidenced by their awareness and adherence to the organization's compliance plan. A compliance plan is the organization's voluntary strategy to ensure that it complies with all requirements and regulations. The healthcare facility must develop a compliance plan after carefully considering and reviewing at least the following:

- State and federal regulations
- HIPAA requirements
- Joint Commission or other accreditation standards
- Medicare rules, including the following:
  - *Conditions of Participation*
  - Coding guidelines
  - Claims-processing guidelines
- Medicaid rules

A great way to begin understanding compliance is to become familiar with the **Office of Inspector General's (OIG's) seven elements** (also called guidances) for a compliance program. HIM managers, as well as any other staff involved in the day-to-day revenue cycle financial operations processes, must be very familiar with the elements that are specific to their healthcare organizations. The OIG's seven elements are listed in figure 3.4; the most recent guidelines, including the 2005 supplement with new OIG recommendations, are available on the OIG website (OIG 2016). The guidelines identify policies and procedures that healthcare organizations should include in their compliance plan. HIM managers must review the guidelines and ensure that their facilities have implemented the policies and procedures in their plan. This process may require updating an existing policy or adopting a new one. HIM managers also may find themselves qualified to assume the role of compliance officer in their healthcare organization. Appendix 2.1 in the online resources shows a sample job description, and appendix 2.2 provides a checklist for monitoring coding compliance.

All departments involved in the revenue cycle process must understand their role in the compliance program and be trained to assist in ensuring that the healthcare facility does not commit fraud. To illustrate the extent to which CMS audits for compliance, table 3.5 lists key monitoring programs and their highlights. Providers need to be aware of these programs and keep abreast of the focus of their audits to ensure that they are not caught unaware of a potential problem that could have been detected and corrected.

Fraud and Abuse

Recent changes to reimbursement have forced healthcare facilities to monitor fraud and abuse more vigilantly. **Fraud** is that which is done erroneously to purposely achieve gain from another.

Figure 3.4. OIG compliance program guidance for hospitals

At a minimum, comprehensive compliance programs should include the following seven elements:

1. The development and distribution of written standards of conduct, as well as written policies and procedures that promote the hospital's commitment to compliance (e.g., by including adherence to compliance as an element in evaluating managers and employees) and that address specific areas of potential fraud, such as claims development and submission processes, code gaming, and financial relationships with physicians and other healthcare professionals;

2. The designation of a chief compliance officer and other appropriate bodies, e.g., a corporate compliance committee, charged with the responsibility of operating and monitoring the compliance program, and who report directly to the CEO and the governing body;

3. The development and implementation of regular, effective education and training programs for all affected employees;

4. The maintenance of a process, such as a hotline, to receive complaints, and the adoption of procedures to protect the anonymity of complainants and to protect whistleblowers from retaliation;

5. The development of a system to respond to allegations of improper/illegal activities and the enforcement of appropriate disciplinary action against employees who have violated internal compliance policies, applicable statutes, regulations or Federal healthcare program requirements;

6. The use of audits and/or other evaluation techniques to monitor compliance and assist in the reduction of identified problem area; and

7. The investigation and remediation of identified systemic problems and the development of policies addressing the non-employment or retention of sanctioned individuals.

Source: Compliance Program Guidance for Hospitals, 63 Fed. Reg, 8987, 8989 (Feb. 23, 1998). For supplementary guidance see Supplemental Compliance Program Guidance for Hospitals, Fed. Reg. 4858-4876 (January 31, 2005).

Table 3.5. Key CMS monitoring programs

Topic	NCCI Edits	MUEs	MR Program	CERT Program	Recovery Audit Program
Providers & Suppliers Impacted are those who submit claims for:	Part B services using HCPCS/CPT codes	Part B services using HCPCS/CPT codes	FFS services & items	FFS services & items	FFS services & items
Medicare Contractor	NCCI Contractor develops the edits; MACs operate the edits	NCCI Contractor develops the edits; MACs operate the edits	MACs ZPICs/PSCs SMRC	CERT RC CERT DC CERT SC	Medicare FFS Recovery Auditors
Claims Impacted	All Part B practitioner, Ambulatory Surgical Center (ASC), and hospital OPPS claims screened	All Part B practitioner, ASC, outpatient hospital, Durable Medical Equipment (DME), and therapy claims screened	Targeted claim review – number varies by MR strategy, or by CMS direction	Limited random claim sample	Widespread or targeted claim review
Prepayment Edit/ Medical Record Review	Yes – tables updated quarterly	Yes – tables updated quarterly	Yes (MACs and ZPICs/PSCs)	No	No
Postpayment Medical Record Review	No	No	Yes	Yes	No – if clear payment error Yes – if likely payment error
Provider Response to Audit Request	N/A	N/A	**Prepayment Review** – Providers must submit medical records to MAC/ZPIC/PSC within 45 calendar days of request. **Postpayment Review** – Providers must submit medical records to the MAC/SMRC within 45 calendar days of the request, 30 calendar days for ZPICs/PSCs*	Providers must submit medical records to the CERT DC within 45 calendar days of the request*	Providers must submit medical records to the Recovery Auditor within 45 calendar days of the request*
Right to Appeal	Yes	Yes	Yes	Yes	Yes

* Extension to submit medical records may be granted
Source: CMS 2015c.

For example, to knowingly and willingly code a patient account to a higher-weighted DRG without supporting documentation to increase reimbursement is fraud. Thus, a hospital would be committing fraud if it falsely assigned all ventilator cases as if every ventilator patient were on the ventilator for over 96 hours through a tracheostomy. **Abuses** are coding errors that occur without intent to defraud the government or other payers (for example, a coding rule was not known or updated or was misused). If a provider routinely uses CPT code 99307 for a nursing facility visit over a period of time and it is later determined that the documentation supports a higher level of visit, code 99308, 99309, or 99310 should have been assigned to those visits.

Fraud and abuse rules and regulations do more than govern a healthcare facility as it relates to reimbursement from Medicare and Medicaid. According to the contracts between state and payer, managed Medicare and managed Medicaid must be treated like traditional Medicare and Medicaid to ensure that benefit coverage to the beneficiary does not change. However, managed Medicare or managed Medicaid may offer additional benefits not traditionally covered by Medicare or Medicaid. Managed Medicare and managed Medicaid payers are required to carry over federal regulatory requirements as well as state Medicaid requirements into the agreement between the payer and the provider. Commercial payers have fraud language in contracts under their billing as well as payment clauses that are based on federal fraud and abuse standards.

Impact of ICD-10 on the Revenue Cycle

ICD-10-CM was adopted by the United States in 2009 and was implemented on October 1, 2015. ICD-10-CM replaces the *ICD-9-CM Diagnostic Index and Tabular (Volumes 1 and 2)*. In addition to the diagnostic codes, the United States has also developed a companion Procedure Coding System, ICD-10-PCS, which replaces ICD-9-CM, volume 3.

Upgrading to ICD-10-CM/PCS has brought many benefits, including increasing the number of codes available for assignment and greatly improving specificity in procedures to include laterality, which accounts for a significant number of new codes. As always, accurate and complete documentation is important to proper code assignment for reimbursement. While the impact of the fully implemented code set was expected to have no net effect on federal reimbursement payments, any bearing on revenue cycle and provider reimbursement remains to be seen.

Patient Safety and Quality Outcomes

Quality care has been a focus in healthcare for at least a century and was the impetus for the formation of many well-known professional organizations, including the American College of Surgeons, the Joint Commission, and the American Health Information Management Association (AHIMA). Numerous iterations of quality and performance improvement activities have evolved into standard-setting and watchdog agencies. Data collection and reporting have become critical and somewhat contentious. CMS has stepped into this arena with the creation of its Hospital Compare website, which allows the general public can look up and compare individual hospitals (CMS 2016b).

Striving for outcomes that reflect high-quality patient care is (or should be) the foundation for decision-making in any healthcare organization. The measurement of these outcomes, whether it is death rates, infection rates, treatment success rates, or some other statistical presentation, has an impact on the organization's ability to recruit and retain talented caregivers, enter into payer contracts, and, ultimately, draw in patients. Therefore, quality outcomes are a revenue cycle issue. While the marketing, physician recruitment, and payer negotiations take place outside a typical revenue cycle team meeting, the team itself must be aware that decisions made to facilitate revenue generation, documentation, and collection must also consider patient satisfaction, safety, quality care, and excellent outcomes.

1. What is the difference between fraud and abuse?

2. List the seven elements of a hospital compliance plan.

Contract Management

In general, a provider is well advised to obtain contracts with a variety of payers. First and foremost, participation in payer plans increases the potential patient pool. Although contract management at the back end can be somewhat cumbersome, it is easier than obtaining preauthorization and payment terms on a case-by-case basis for out-of-plan patients. In addition, the maintenance of contracts establishes a foundation for financial projections. When providers can confidently estimate potential reimbursement levels, they are better able to predict payer mix and forecast financial results for specific scenarios.

Contract Basics

All written business contracts contain some standard provisions. The body of the contract spells out the relationship between the parties and their specific obligations in fulfillment of the purpose of the agreement. The administrative terms contain, but are not limited to, the duration of the agreement, the law governing the agreement, the circumstances under which the contract may be terminated and what actions must take place to terminate early, official contact information for the parties, and a clause absolving the parties from negligence in the presence of circumstances beyond their control (force majeure). Finally, all written contracts end with the signatures of the individuals authorized to make the contract on behalf of the parties. Contracts may also begin with a series of introductory statements identifying the parties and recitations outlining the purpose of the contract. The body or the attached rate schedule of a managed care contract will detail financial terms, including the requirements that must be met by the provider to be reimbursed for services by the payer.

Financial projections must be incorporated into contract negotiations. If a payer is to be given a discount on charges, then the impact of that discount on revenue and thus net income must be estimated in the context of all payers, as illustrated in table 3.6.

The main issue in contract negotiation is understanding both the marketplace and the cost to provide service in that marketplace. To restate the obvious, increasing the volume of a service provided at a loss will not generate profit. The actual contract itself will contain the reimbursements

Table 3.6. Example of the impact of discounts on net income

Chest x-Ray (Cost per Case = $125)	Estimated Number of Cases	Revenue at $180.18 Charge per Case
Payer 1 reimburses 70% of charges	350	$ 44,144.10
Payer 2 reimburses a flat $100 rate	250	$ 25,000.00
Payer 3 reimburses 100% of charges	300	$ 54,054.00
Self-pay and charity care pay 10% of charges	100	$ 1,801.80
Total	1,000	$124,999.90

Cost calculation: Cost per Case × Total No. of Patients = $125 × 1,000 = $125,000
Charge calculation: (350 × 0.70X) + (100 × 250) + (300X) + (100 × 0.10X) = $125,000
To cover costs, the facility must charge at least $180.18 per case (X = 180.18).

for specific items, procedures, and services. It is important to review the reimbursements not just in the context of cost but also in the listing of reimbursable services. If a service is not included in the contract, and there is no general provision for reimbursement of unlisted services, then the provider cannot expect to be paid for those services. For example, the provider may have a thriving physical therapy department. However, if physical therapy is not listed in the contract, the patient covered by this particular payer must self-pay for physical therapy services.

In addition to the reimbursement specifics, a payer contract includes abundant administrative language. This language covers the relationship between the provider and the payer, the duration of the agreement, payment terms, documentation requirements, the auditability of the claims and underlying documentation, the jurisdiction and methodology of dispute resolution, and any other requirements that the payer and provider deem necessary.

Specific Contract Clauses

Ambiguity in contract language makes contract management difficult, if not impossible. For example, assume that the contract specifies the use of CMS IPPS DRGs as the basis for the inpatient fee schedule and lists those DRGs in the schedule. The contract was written in 2012 and continues to 2017. Without specifying that the fee schedule would be amended annually to reflect the appropriate DRGs, how would reimbursement be affected in 2015 with the implementation of ICD-10-CM/PCS?

Additionally, parties to the contract need to ensure that appropriate audit periods are reciprocal and are included in the billing and payment clause within the body of the contract. Several states have managed care regulations that govern look-back or audit periods, which range can from 12 to 24 months. It is important to know your state's managed care and health maintenance organization (HMO) regulations, which are designed to help protect the provider. Timely filing deadlines (which range from 30 to 365 days) and clean-claims parameters, including the payer-specific definition for clean claims, are also found within the billing and payment clause and should be reviewed against federal and state regulations. The billing and payment clause is also where time frames for reimbursement should be addressed. The discount should become null and void if the payer does not pay on time, according to the terms spelled out in the specific contract.

State regulations generally apply to fully insured patients only, but self-insured patients can be included in these provisions during the contract negotiations process. Part of the negotiation process is ensuring that there are not two different provisions within the contract for the patient accounting services, care management, and PFS departments to differentiate.

Other clauses that will significantly affect the healthcare facility's reimbursement are new technology and new services rate amendments and carve-out and materiality clauses. New technology and new services would be covered if the rate amendment stipulates that when the provider brings on a new service, whether or not it includes a technology component, the payer will reimburse a specific percentage for the new services until the parties come to agreement on new rates. Generally, the payer will specify a time frame in which the new rate must be negotiated and will typically want 30 to 60 days' advance notice that the new service or technology will be offered.

A carve-out clause is meant to protect the provider from a payer deciding to outsource the case management and payment of a service line (such as physical therapy) after the agreement has been signed. The carve-out clause says that a payer may outsource the case management and payment functions, but the provider's reimbursement will be based on the terms outlined in the rate schedule in the full agreement.

The intent of materiality language in a contract is to protect the provider financially if a payer, especially a nationally based payer, gives a 30-day notice of a change in policy that affects reimbursement. Providers conduct financial analyses at the point of contract-rate negotiations, which lock in the agreement's financial value to the provider. If a materiality provision is not included, the provider essentially allows the payer unilateral ability to change the financial value of the contract; the provider may be locked in an initial term or not have a "without cause" clause, and therefore be left with no recourse. The materiality clause is generally needed in two sections of the contract: the case-management section to cover inpatient services, and the billing and payment section to cover outpatient and all other services. The intent of the material provision can also be covered in the miscellaneous section under amendments by simply saying the contract cannot be amended without the written consent of both parties. However, this simple addition to the miscellaneous or amendment provisions is not an easy point to win during a negotiation.

Additional protection against financial disadvantage must be requested in the term and termination provision as well as in the arbitration provision (if such a provision is in the contract). Many payers expect a provider to sign a multiyear contract and give up the without-cause clause until the term of the initial contract ends, which makes the arbitration provision important to review. If a payer asks to exclude a without-cause clause, a provider should use that as a deal-breaker during negotiations whenever possible. Once the new contract period begins sans a without-cause clause, the provider is locked in with only the arbitration clause to use as protection if the payer defaults on timely payment. Even when invoking the material breach clause, providers generally must rely on the arbitration clause if the payer does not remedy the breach within the specified time frame. If possible, providers may want to exclude an arbitration clause from the contract. The absence of an arbitration clause preserves the provider's right to file a lawsuit and does not mean that the provider cannot ask the payer to mediate or arbitrate an issue. If an arbitration clause must go into the agreement, providers should review it thoroughly with legal counsel to understand when the material breach clause will allow the provider to get out of the contract, regardless of the status of the arbitration.

Retroactive denials occur when the provider contacts the payer prior to providing a service, obtains an authorization code, and then is later denied payment. One reason that payment might be denied is for lack of medical necessity, as determined upon retroactive review. Another reason is that the subscriber may have canceled the contract with the payer. If the diagnostic information is conveyed to the payer in advance and the correct service is rendered, then retroactive denials should not take place. The process for obtaining prior authorization should be spelled out in the contract, and that process becomes an agreement to pay for that service according to the terms. A discussion of denials is included in chapter 7.

The payer is likely to deny reimbursement for any service that it deems medically unnecessary. However, the physician may disagree. Such a dispute may be due to the physician's failure to communicate the correct diagnostic profile or rule-out diagnoses, or it could arise because the payer relies on a canned list of rationales for reimbursing for a service; regardless, the fact is that the provider is at risk to lose the reimbursement if the issue is not resolved. It would not be unusual for the physician to receive payment for an office visit while the ancillary testing provider is denied payment for the service that same physician ordered during the visit. Operationally, the provider can publish order sheets that require the physician to specify the medical reason for every test or therapy. Contractually, the provider can protect itself by inserting appeal clauses that rely on a third party to determine whether the service was medically necessary.

One common reason for denials is that the provider failed to submit a clean claim. Therefore, the contract should define what a clean claim means to the payer. Generally, the clean-claims definition is based on federal or state (managed Medicaid or state HMO or managed care) regulations. The payer will generally have a billing and claims submission policy, which should be expressly referenced in the contract. PFS should review the policy before the provider accepts the terms.

A "most-favored nation" clause means payer A dictates in its contract that the provider may not negotiate terms with other payers that are more favorable than the terms in payer A's contract.

This clause is restrictive to the provider and limits its ability to negotiate in the marketplace. These types of clauses are difficult to administer and enforce (Cleverley et al. 2011, 149). As such, many states have deemed this type of clause obsolete because it restricts fair trade between the providers and payers.

Providers should "prohibit silent PPO arrangements" (Cleverley et al. 2011, 149–150), in which payers have arrangements with subcontracted providers so that all discounts flow through to the subcontractor. Unless silent PPO arrangements are specifically prohibited in the payer contract, the provider may be at risk for allowing such discounts to all of the payer's subcontractors. These silent arrangements should be carefully reviewed and possibly prohibited by the provider or organization. The provider should request a list of affiliates, or clients, as an addendum or exhibit to the main contract. The addendum should include language that allows the provider to request that such a list be shared with the provider within 30 days of the request.

The phrase *establish ability to recover payment after termination* refers to limiting the period after termination during which the terms of the contract still apply. Allowing the maintenance of contract terms for an extended period of time may not be beneficial to the provider. It is important to review state regulations, which may impose on providers additional mandatory time periods to continue to see patients past the contractually agreed-upon termination date. In New Jersey, for example, state HMO regulation requires providers to see fully insured patients for 120 days past the contract termination date, essentially extending the termination period and, therefore, the provider's obligation with the payer an additional 120 days for fully insured patients.

Providers should *preserve the ability to be paid for services*. The Medicare Advanced Beneficiary Notice (ABN) is a notice to the patient that certain services are not covered by Medicare. The provider cannot bill the patient for noncovered services if the ABN has not been signed. For commercial payers, no such requirement exists. However, if the payer contract specifies that the provider agrees to accept payer reimbursement, the provider may not be able to bill the patient for denied services. The provider can request that the patient sign a self-pay waiver that outlines services that may not be covered by insurance. The signed waiver can serve as acknowledgment that the payer deemed a service experimental or noncovered. It is important to review the hold-harmless language in a contract during negotiation to ensure that the payer acknowledges in what cases the healthcare facility will balance-bill the patient regardless of benefit coverage. Generally, the payer will not reimburse the provider if the patient, the payer's member, could have waited for their referring provider to get the necessary authorization to have the service. Standard hold-harmless language says the provider cannot balance bill the patient in this scenario. During the negotiation process, it is important to ensure that the payer acknowledges that the hospital can balance bill the member when the member wants to be seen and agrees to self-pay. The ABN and self-pay waivers are discussed in detail in chapter 4.

Finally, providers should minimize health plan rate differentials, which refers to the goal to "establish a rate structure for all plans and grant discounts for administrative efficiencies only" (Cleverley et al. 2011, 151). With the volume of data available these days and the ability to benchmark against Medicare effectively, achievement of this goal is complex but possible.

Health Insurance Exchange and Federal Facilitated Exchange

Provisions of the Affordable Care Act (ACA) began to roll out in 2012. The health insurance exchange (HIX) that began operations on January 1, 2014, was one of the largest and most significant components of the ACA. With the creation of the HIX, many underinsured and uninsured Americans were able to go online and purchase insurance with federal subsidies to offset the monthly premiums offered to some people based on income levels. The plans are a tiered system. Bronze is the basic package and has more out-of-pocket expenses while charging a lower premium. Premiums for silver, gold, and platinum plans increase incrementally, respectively, but include additional coverage with less out-of-pocket expense.

The HIX website for the federal facilitated exchanges (FFEs) also allow users to assess whether they qualify for their state's Medicaid program and automatically sends their information to the state for processing. States that agreed to accept federal funds to expand their Medicaid program have seen a reduction in charity care and an increase in Medicaid or managed Medicaid, as most states have rolled their Medicaid program into managed Medicaid. This is good financial news for hospitals that may have been getting less than 10 cents on the dollar for charity care but are now getting closer to 20 cents on the dollar for Medicaid. Hospitals need to conduct their own financial impact analysis of managed Medicaid as each facility's charity care and Medicaid dollars vary. States that chose not to be a part of the FFE and instead opted to develop their state-based HIX have tiers and plan designs that meet the minimum threshold for coverage as defined in the ACA. The states decide whether to set the minimum coverage threshold higher than the FFE.

The ACA does not allow any insurance company to discriminate on the basis of an individual's pre-existing conditions; they must cover members who have such conditions. The ACA also prohibits lifetime maximums in which a chronically ill person could reach the maximum allowable insurance benefits and no longer qualify for coverage. The ACA has allowed for additional access to care, which financially benefits all providers, including hospitals, because fewer patients are now uninsured or underinsured.

When conducting financial analyses related to contract negotiations, it is important to determine how much of the patient population is HIX by payer, especially if the hospital negotiated a lower rate for HIX members with a payer. HIX payers tend to have narrower networks, so verifying whether the hospital is a participating provider and at what tiered level with the HIX plans is crucial in determining financial impact. The implementation of federal and state Medicare and Medicaid ACOs as well as the creation of other P4P and quality and patient-safety programs, such as the Medicaid DSRIP, are all due to the ACA. Being able to see the financial impact of a regulation as far-reaching and significant as the ACA has been and will continue to be a critical challenge to all providers as financial data is monitored through revenue cycle management.

HIM's Role in Data Management

As previously stated, an HIM manager is typically not directly responsible for cost accounting. However, HIM managers need a basic understanding of cost concepts, including how costs are allocated, and a general understanding of how charges are determined; such knowledge will improve the manager's performance in the budget process and in participation in revenue cycle management. The HIM role, then, is generally to ensure the quality of coded data and support the analysis of that data (Davis 2005).

Data Quality

Coded clinical data are the primary contribution of the HIM department to the payer negotiation process. An accurate postdischarge database is critical to developing volume measures and calculating a CMI. On the billing side, HIM can also play a role in charge description master (CDM) maintenance, as discussed in chapter 5. Ensuring that CPT/HCPCS codes are current and properly used is an important part of CDM maintenance. Further, the review and validation of abstracted data, such as patient discharge dispositions, further assist in maintaining the integrity of the data and supporting the revenue cycle. For example, statistics related to volume, payer mix, and DRG are used to support analysis of payer contracts.

Providing and Analyzing Data

Because HIM generates coded data, HIM managers are often called on to report on and explain these data. This secondary use of data is an important HIM responsibility. Standard reports in the abstracting or financial system allow users to pull data based on ICD-10-CM or CPT/HCPCS codes.

Ad-hoc or routine custom reporting can generally be arranged either through the information technology (IT) department or with a plug-in report writer. It is best practice is for HIM managers to have access to report writers and be adequately trained in their use.

Even if HIM department personnel do not have access to the reporting modules, they are often called on to provide information regarding the diagnosis or procedure codes that would yield the data required for a particular project. For example, if the hospital's administration is analyzing use of endoscopies, the procedure codes that reflect this type of procedure might be required. HIM department directors, although not routinely required to code records, should be sufficiently familiar with coding and coded data to ensure that the HIM department can efficiently provide this type of support.

In addition to consulting on the codes needed for a project, HIM personnel may perform the analysis itself. Health information administration students learn data analysis skills through the study of statistics and research. A practical application of those skills is in the analysis of coded data to provide the hospital's administration and other departments with needed information, not just data.

Special Considerations for Specific Practice Settings

The goal in any practice setting is to ensure that the provider is able to attract sufficient volume at reimbursement rates that, in aggregate, enable the provider to achieve its strategic goals and objectives. However, the perspectives vary a bit depending on the specific setting.

Inpatient Settings

On the inpatient side, reimbursement issues vary by setting. Even the prospective payment systems vary in the ways they are reimbursed. For example, IPPS pays a specific rate for the entire visit whereas IRPPS reimburses on a per diem basis, even though both systems use a calculated DRG to determine the reimbursement rate. When negotiating contracts with payers, the accurate projection of the payer mix and an understanding of the fully allocated cost of providing services are critical. It may be necessary to consider factors that skew the costs of providing services, such as high-dollar pharmaceuticals and other supplies, separately from per diem payments.

Outpatient Settings

Although the costs for outpatient services can be easier to calculate than inpatient costs, the volume of cases and the complexity of the coding and billing rules in outpatient settings make outpatient reimbursement potentially more difficult. Understanding the marketplace and the competition is critical. A major financial risk in providing outpatient services is that services ordered by a physician may not be reimbursable by the patient's particular plan. For example, just because a physician ordered a test does not mean the payer will pay for that test. Outpatient providers should make every effort to ensure that their services are included in specific contracts and that prices are set to properly allow for variations in reimbursement.

Physician Practices

Physicians are in the unenviable position of being subject to payer rate setting as well as pressure from hospital providers to deliver volume. Some physicians may choose to forego participation in payer plans, including Medicare. In such cases, the physician is an out-of-network or non-par (par is shorthand for participating) provider, which may raise the patient's obligation for payment. Other physicians choose to associate with a payer or hospital provider as an employee. Physicians negotiating an employee contract should take care to ensure that they are able to maintain a private practice at the same time, should they wish to do so.

Some physicians desire to merge their practices with or have them acquired by larger physician groups or a hospital. These mergers and acquisitions are happening more frequently as smaller practices and independent physicians experience the financial impact of meaningful use, Medicare ACOs, PCMHs, and the general reduction in reimbursement from payers. Physician practices are generally in separate facilities from hospitals; however, from a revenue cycle standpoint, these relationships need to be monitored carefully and their costs and expenses tied in to the hospital's finances when overall costs are reviewed and payer contracts are negotiated.

Check Your Understanding 3.3.

1. What is the relationship between charges and reimbursement?

2. What is an RVU and why is it important?

3. What is the main goal of contract negotiation from the provider's perspective?

References

42 CFR 412.160: Definitions for the hospital value-based purchasing (VBP) program. 2014 (Aug 22).

Butler, M. CMS to End Meaningful Use in 2016. 2016 (January). *Journal of AHIMA.* http://journal.ahima .org/2016/01/13/cms-to-end-meaningful-use-in-2016/.

Centers for Medicare and Medicaid Services (CMS). 2016a. Medicare Provider Reimbursement Manual, Part 1, Chapter 22. 2202.4. https://www.cms.gov/Regulations-and-Guidance/Guidance/Manuals/Paper -Based-Manuals-Items/CMS021929.html.

Centers for Medicare and Medicaid Services (CMS). 2016b. Hospital Compare. http://www.medicare.gov /hospitalcompare/search.html.

Centers for Medicare and Medicaid Services (CMS). 2015a. Hospital Outpatient PPS. https://www.cms.gov /Medicare/Medicare-Fee-for-Service-Payment/HospitalOutpatientPPS/index.html.

Centers for Medicare and Medicaid Services (CMS). 2015b. Inpatient Psychiatric Facility PPS. https:?// www.cms.gov/Medicare/Medicare-Fee-for-Service-Payment/InpatientPsychFacilPPS/index.html.

Centers for Medicare and Medicaid Services (CMS). 2013. Inpatient Rehabilitation Facility PPS. https:// www.cms.gov/Medicare/Medicare-Fee-for-Service-Payment/InpatientRehabFacPPS/index.html.

Centers for Medicare and Medicaid Services (CMS). 2015c. Medicare Claim Review Programs. https://www .cms.gov/Outreach-and-Education/Medicare-Learning-Network-MLN/MLNProducts/downloads /MCRP_Booklet.pdf.

Cleverley, W.O., P.H. Song, and J.O. Cleverley. 2011. Revenue determination. Chapter 6 in *Essentials of Health Care Finance.* Sudbury, MA: Jones and Bartlett.

Davis, N. 2005. Cost accounting. Unit 3 in *Essentials of Healthcare Finance: A Workbook for Health Information Managers.* Chicago, AHIMA.

Hazelwood, A.C. and C.A. Venable. 2014. Reimbursement methodologies. Chapter 6 in *Health Information Management Technology: An Applied Approach,* Fourth Edition. Ed. N. Sayles. Chicago: AHIMA.

Office of Inspector General (OIG). 1998. Compliance program guidance for hospitals. *Federal Register* 63(35):8988–8989.

Office of Inspector General (OIG). 2005. Supplementary guidance. *Federal Register* 70(19):4858–4876.

Office of Inspector General (OIG). 2016. Compliance Guidance. http://oig.hhs.gov/compliance/compliance -guidance/index.asp.

Additional Resources

Casto, A. and E. Forrestal. 2015. *Principles of Healthcare Reimbursement,* 5th ed. Chicago: AHIMA.

Centers for Medicare and Medicaid Services. 2016. Guide to the Health Insurance Marketplace. https:// www.healthcare.gov/quick-guide/one-page-guide-to-the-marketplace.

Trela, P. 2007. IRF PPS coding challenges. *Journal of AHIMA* 78(5):70–71.

Patient Access

Learning Objectives

- Evaluate the flow of the patient registration process.
- Identify the key revenue cycle data collected at patient access points.
- Review patient records for duplicate medical record numbers.
- Analyze the insurance verification process for compliance with best practices.
- Examine the reimbursement issues that arise from incomplete verification of insurance.
- Compare and contrast the registration processing of a fully insured patient versus a patient who self-pays or is underinsured.

Key Terms

- Account number
- Admissions
- Advance beneficiary notice (ABN)
- Centralized model
- Decentralized model
- Emergency Medical Treatment and Active Labor Act (EMTALA)
- Encounter

- Government payers
- Hybrid model
- Inpatient
- Master patient index (MPI)
- Medical identity theft
- Medical record number
- MPI cleanup
- Outpatient
- Patient access

- Patient identification number
- Patient registration
- Red Flag Rules
- Registration
- Self-pay
- Uniform Hospital Discharge Data Set (UHDDS)
- Visit

The primary purpose of this chapter is to convey that the collection, verification, and recording of patient data at the point of entry into the facility is critical to efficient and effective revenue cycle management. Realizing that there are many variations in the process due to the facility needs and clinical urgency of the encounter, the descriptions in this chapter focus on the control points rather than an ideal process flow. Further, there are various facility-specific terms for many of the concepts and activities described in this chapter. To avoid confusion, generic terms are used throughout this chapter, with the intent of providing sufficient description for readers to connect what happens at their facilities with what is being described herein.

As described in chapter 1, patient access is the first step on the journey to a clean claim. **Patient access** is an individual or department of individuals charged with the responsibility of collecting data that initiates the documentation for the patient encounter, a process called **registration**. Thus, patient access is variously called **patient registration** or **admissions**. The data collected or initiated by patient access are critical to the accurate accumulation of patient data and the timely processing of an error-free claim. This chapter discusses the relationship of patient access to the revenue cycle.

Data Flow

There are multiple steps in the registration process, and all of them must take place at some point in the patient encounter. In emergent care, collection of some patient demographic and clinical data is necessary for triage; however, the collection of financial data would likely take place later in the encounter, after the medical screening examination (CFR 2004).

Critical Data

There are four types of data collected during a patient encounter: patient identification, administrative data, financial data, and clinical data. Collection of the first three types of data is initiated or completed by patient access, and these data then flow directly to the bill. Patient identification data, such as name, address, and date of birth, serve to distinguish one patient from another and to facilitate matching when data are transmitted from one system to another. Administrative data, such as patient identification and account numbers, provide the facility with the ability to cumulate both billing data and clinical data associated with patient services. Financial data collected by patient access are related to the patient's method of payment. Additional financial data pertaining to individual services are recorded in the service areas. Clinical data are recorded by clinicians and other patient service staff as services are provided. For example, a physician records an order for a blood test, and laboratory staff record laboratory service data when the test is performed. The order, test results, and associated billing data are linked to the patient by the patient identification and account numbers. Table 4.1 summarizes the four data types discussed in this section.

Organizational Issues

The processing of the patient's registration may be performed in a centralized department or in a decentralized manner by the clinical departments. Inpatient registrations are usually processed by a centralized department; in contrast, outpatient services often have individual registration activities. Table 4.2 summarizes several different possible organizational structures.

There are advantages and disadvantages to each registration scenario described in table 4.2, and there is no universally right way to organize the function.

In a **centralized model**, the registrars report to the patient access department and generally are located in one space or a limited number of spaces. Centralization facilitates training, data collection consistency, and compliance, but it may decrease flexibility in the registration process. For example, some clinical areas may have unique registration requirements. Should those areas complete the registration process themselves or should the patient access department require all registrars to be trained on all registrations? An alternative is to create registration specialties in the patient access department, which may inhibit the ability of the department to flex staff into different areas.

In a fully **decentralized model**, registrars report to the department for which they are registering and may be located in that department. Decentralization facilitates flexibility in the registration process, but it may increase inconsistency in data collection. It also affects patient flow. If patients are visiting more than one department in the same day, what impact will that have on the registration process? Will registration practices vary among departments? Will the patient need to register multiple times? How will the Advanced Beneficiary Notice (discussed later in

Table 4.1. Four types of data collected during a patient encounter

Data Type	Overview	Role of patient access or other revenue cycle team member
Patient identification	Patient demographics Required data includes race/ethnicity, date of birth	Collection, verification, and recording
Administrative	Patient identification numbers Patient account numbers Dates of service	Assignment of numbers and beginning service dates during the registration process
Financial	How the bill for services rendered will be paid The charges for the services rendered The record of billing and payment Codes assigned to clinical documentation	Collection, verification, and recording of insurance data. Codes for admitting diagnosis and reason for admission may be assigned by patient access. Codes for specific outpatient services may be assigned by patient access. Completed services are recorded by the area rendering the service. Records of billing and payment are maintained by patient financial services. Codes assigned at the completion of services for data and billing purposes are generally assigned in HIM or the clinical department rendering the service.
Clinical	Documentation of services rendered	Recorded in the clinical areas.

Table 4.2. Control over registration

Organization	Registrars Report to	Locations
Centralized registration	Patient access department	A limited number of locations—for example, one location for the emergency department and another for all other types of patients. Facility may carve out a location for ambulatory surgery patients or provide access points in different buildings or on different campuses.
Centralized control / decentralized registration	Patient access department	Separate registration points for each service department—for example, ambulatory surgery, emergency, inpatient, laboratory, radiology, therapy.
Decentralized control / decentralized registration	Service department	Some patients, such as inpatients, may come through the patient access department, but service departments maintain their own registration staff.

this chapter) be developed? How many registrars will each department need to ensure coverage for illness and vacation?

In a **hybrid model**, all registrars report to patient access, but they are located in the departments they serve. This model takes advantage of the training, data collection consistency, and compliance of the centralized model as well as the specialization of the decentralized model.

This model also enables the patient access department to flex staff where they are needed for coverage. The challenges with this model involves the relationship between patient access, which supervises the registrars, and the departments in which the registrars are located. If the clinical department is not satisfied with the work of the registrar, what steps should the patient access department take to resolve the issue? How will the patient access department supervise the registrars efficiently, particularly if registrars are located in different buildings?

The impact on patient satisfaction of each scenario depends on the specific implementation and leadership within the organization. From a revenue cycle perspective, the primary goal of patient access is to ensure data quality and identify reimbursement issues. Each facility must decide what structure best suits its needs and proceed accordingly.

Patient Identification and Administrative Data

Patient identification and demographics and administrative data enable the provider to distinguish one patient from another and to accurately document multiple encounters by the same patient. Some administrative data, such as primary language and religion, enable us to provide better patient care and other services.

Pre-existing Identification Numbers

All patient encounters must be easily accessible for patient care, retrospective review, and release of information. The easiest way to link encounters is through the use of a **patient identification number** (also known as a **medical record number**, health record number, history number, or chart number) that is assigned to the patient at the first encounter and then used to identify the patient through all subsequent encounters. Typically, the assignment of the number is automatic when the registrar indicates a new patient is being registered. This unit-numbering system lends itself well to subsequent filing in the health information management (HIM) department as well as the compilation of data in an electronic health record (EHR).

For the unit-numbering system to work, the registrar must first make sure that the patient is not already in the system. Once the registrar verifies a patient is new, he or she must then enter all of that patient's data correctly during registration. For example, when Arturo Bennini comes to registration for the initial encounter, the registrar must enter the patient name correctly and verify the patient's demographic data—usually by reviewing documentation such as a driver's license. If Mr. Bennini returns to the facility, the ease of finding his previously assigned number depends in part on how many patients named Arturo Bennini have been registered at the facility. The registrar should be able to scan a master patient index list of those with the surname Bennini that also includes, at a minimum, first names, street addresses, and dates of birth. Thus, the key differences between same-named patients are clearly visible and the risk of incorrectly selecting the identification number for another patient named Bennini is minimized. Several challenges arise in the selection of an existing record:

- **Misspelled names:** If the surname in the original registration is entered as Benini, it will be difficult for the registrar to find the original record. Searching on the first few letters of the name—in this example, *Ben*—can help alleviate this problem. Many systems include a phonetic feature that lists potential records by how they sound rather than how they are spelled. Thus, Benini and Bennini would both appear on the phonetic list.
- **Patient denial of prior admission:** For a variety of reasons, some patients may not remember a previous encounter at the facility. They may not associate registration for laboratory tests with the registration for an inpatient visit. Perhaps the previous registration took place in a different location or the facility has changed names. Other patients may have

nefarious reasons for not identifying a previous encounter. For example, a patient might owe a balance on the bill for a previous encounter or attempt to receive care using another person's identity. Therefore, the registrar should always search for a previous encounter, even if the patient states that he or she has never been to the facility before.

- **Previous registration under a different name:** There are many reasons why a patient's name might change, including marriage, divorce, and adoption. A newborn may be registered under the mother's maiden name but return under a different name at a later date. Inquiry about any previous names used and asking whether a child was born at that hospital can direct the search for previous encounters.

When a registrar fails to identify a previous encounter, a new record is created and a new medical record number is assigned to the patient. In this scenario, one patient has multiple medical record numbers or what is known as a duplicate medical record number.

Duplicate Medical Record Numbers

Duplicate medical record numbers are problematic. Previous clinical encounters will not be displayed in the patient's record, which may have a negative impact on patient care. For this reason, duplicate medical record numbers are a patient safety issue. Previous account balances also will not be associated with the duplicate number, and the encounters will be filed differently and will not be properly identified for release-of-information purposes. Furthermore, duplicate medical record numbers corrupt the **master patient index (MPI)**, the key to locating patient records by searching on a specific field. The MPI is used by the patient access department to identify previous encounters and by the HIM department to find records for processing. It is also used by anyone who needs to access a patient's health record, including caregivers. Finally, as the index to all records, the MPI is accessed by electronic queries when data are pulled by analysts. Therefore, the accuracy of the MPI is of critical importance to the integrity of the organization's data and information governance programs.

Duplicate medical record numbers may be identified by patient access at registration, by patient accounting during billing, or by the HIM department during a targeted audit for cleanup of the MPI. Most often, the HIM department is responsible for actively searching for duplicate medical record numbers and resolving the problem.

MPI Cleanups

The purpose of an **MPI cleanup** is to identify and correct duplicate medical record numbers. The correction process includes the merging of the duplicate records so that the patient is correctly listed under only one number. This merge must include not only the electronic listing but also any associated electronic records and any paper documentation. Although the activity of locating and correcting the error is generally an HIM function, all relevant areas of the facility must be notified so that any ancillary records can also be amended. MPI cleanup can therefore be a labor-intensive and costly process.

The notification of ancillary areas regarding health-record merges is critical for the proper identification and tracking of clinical results. It cannot be assumed that ancillary clinical systems, such as laboratory and pharmacy, are interfaced to automatically handle merged records. Some systems may need to be manually corrected by the ancillary area. A duplicate health record number can lead to duplicate charges on multiple accounts, which, in turn, can result in claims denials for duplicate charges and may trigger a payer audit. Therefore, patient accounting services must be notified of MPI cleanup to ensure that billing issues are resolved.

The first step in MPI cleanup is to identify potential duplicate records. The easiest method uses matching software that compares key fields in patient accounts to identify duplicates. Some financial and clinical operations systems include this software in their HIM module. If the system does not include matching software, the facility should consider purchasing it or retain a vendor to perform the matching function routinely. Otherwise, the search for duplicate medical record numbers will be tedious, time-consuming, and prone to error. If MPI cleanup is attempted without customized support, MPI data can be queried for duplicate Social Security numbers. Additional queries may include date of birth and, of course, last name.

Once a potential duplicate has been identified, the patient records must be reviewed to determine whether the records, in fact, represent the same individual. Key fields that can be compared include Social Security number, date of birth, and name. Patient insurance and personal identification documentation is most helpful; copies of photo identification are particularly useful. Any variation in data between accounts must be validated before a decision can be made to merge records. Figure 4.1 shows an example of a duplicate record review sheet, which is also available in the online materials.

Figure 4.1. Sample duplicate health record number review sheet

MPI Analysis		
Health Record #1		**Health Record #2**
	Social Security Number	
	Date of Birth	
	Gender	
	Last Name	
	First Name	
	Middle Name	
	Also known as (AKA)	
STOP! If all of the above fields match, and the patient's ID matches, merge the accounts.		
	Address 1	
	Address 2	
	City	
	State	
	Zip	

Disposition:

    Not Merged—referred to patient registration for further analysis

    Not Merged—confirmed different patients

    Merged   Initial and Date

        Records merged in system   _____

        Records renumbered in file room   _____

        Patient Access notified   _____

        Notice sent to ancillary departments _____

        Merge Log updated   _____

If medical record numbers are deemed duplicates, the patient records associated with those numbers can be merged. Merging involves the following:

- Electronically combining the records, which is usually a menu item in the HIM module
- If applicable, manually relabeling the file or folder housing paper records with the duplicate number
- Modifying, as needed, any chart-tracking, deficiency, or other relevant HIM software
- Notifying all relevant departments in the facility, as noted earlier

Note that the analysis that led to the merging of records must be documented to provide a record of the rationale for the action. Even when software support is available to search for potential duplicate medical record numbers, it is only by investigating that the health records can be matched.

Ideally, there should be an audit trail noting the merge in the MPI. In other words, the user should be able to see that there were multiple records at one time and that they have been merged. Since duplicate health record numbers may not be discovered until after information has been released or bills have been dropped and paid, the audit trail provides a historical record of activity under the health record number that now no longer exists. There needs to be some shortcut to finding the reason why a particular number seems to have "disappeared." Although most duplicates will likely merge into a record under the same name, making it fairly evident why the merge occurred, there will be enough merges that involve name changes to justify the routine documentation of the audit trail. No health record number, once assigned, should ever "disappear." The MPI should direct the user to the merged record. Whether or not the system appropriately refers the user, the HIM department should maintain an accessible list of all merged records.

Routine audits are one way to identify duplicate health record numbers. In the normal course of business, duplicates may be reported by ancillary areas, patient access, patient accounting, or even the patient. As such, the HIM department must have a method by which reported instances of duplicate medical record numbers are evaluated and a policy to standardize the decision process. (Several related AHIMA Practice Briefs are found in the online material for this book.) Duplicate medical record numbers represent a risk under the Red Flags Rule (discussed later in this chapter); therefore, a link to that risk management policy should be easily accessible and appropriate actions clearly defined.

In the risk management policy, the number of individuals who have the access and authority to merge medical record numbers must be extremely limited. A merge typically cannot be "undone," and it has potential financial consequences for the patient, such as linking balances due. Therefore, the authority to merge records should reside with an individual of sufficient departmental and organizational level of management to ensure that the function is carried out properly. For example, a clerical person may analyze the records and recommend the merge, but it should not be carried out until an appropriate supervisor approves the request. Such an approval process serves to prevent inappropriate merging.

Technology that facilitates patient identification of returning patients is being introduced. Some hospitals use electronic biometric hand scanners to identify returning patients. New patients can opt into this electronic security measure to protect their confidential information from identity theft and help the hospital prevent insurance fraud. At the time of opt-in, the patient's palm is scanned and the patient's identification is scrutinized. For subsequent visits, no identification paperwork is needed at registration; the patient's health record is located on completion of the palm scan.

Duplicate Account Numbers

In addition to identifying or assigning a medical record number at registration, patient access also assigns a number to the encounter: the **account number**, also called the financial (FIN) number, visit number, or encounter number. All clinical and financial activity associated with a particular encounter is connected to the account number. Although a patient ideally has only one medical record number, the patient can have an unlimited number of account numbers—one for each encounter.

There are many different types of encounters between a patient and a facility. The number and variety depend on the nature of the facility and the services it provides. The terms *encounter* and *visit* are often used interchangeably to describe an episode of care—for example, a physician visit/encounter with a patient, a laboratory visit/encounter for bloodwork. Further, one patient may receive many services from multiple departments on the same day of service. How we capture these relationships at patient registration affects the billing for these services later. To illustrate, we present the following, for which we offer these definitions:

- Encounter: Direct personal contact between a registered outpatient and a clinician or other health care professional for the diagnosis and treatment of an illness or injury from the beginning of a specific group of services to the end of those services.
- Visit: The services provided to a patient by a particular provider or service department during the course of an encounter.
- Outpatient: Any patient who is not an inpatient. Typically, the visit takes place in one calendar day or less than 24 hours, but some visits, such as observation status, can last longer.
- Inpatient: A patient who is admitted to a hospital.

It is important to understand how a facility organizes its patient services so that account numbers are assigned correctly and patient services are billed correctly. A patient generally has one account number per encounter. However, an encounter may have multiple visits. Figure 4.2 offers examples of different ways that a facility might organize its services and accounts.

As illustrated in figure 4.2, the determination of how to organize the patient into a specific account is complicated and goes beyond the assignment of an account number by patient access. For example, the merging of two accounts after discharge might be done by either patient accounting or the HIM department. As with merging medical record numbers, both the criteria and responsibility for merging patient accounts must be clearly delineated. The decision whether to merge two or more accounts should be based on the payer's reimbursement criteria. Medicare requires merging of hospital outpatient accounts into acute care inpatient accounts when the two visits are related or are presumed to be related. This requirement applies to diagnostic services rendered within three days of the inpatient visit and nondiagnostic services provided within three days of the inpatient visit. However, if the hospital can demonstrate that the nondiagnostic services are unrelated to the inpatient visit, the accounts do not have to be merged. Effectively, the merging of an outpatient account into an acute care inpatient account means that Medicare will not pay the facility separately for the outpatient account because, under Medicare, the diagnosis-related group (DRG)–based payment is deemed to have covered both the outpatient and inpatient accounts (CMS 2014a).

Check Your Understanding 4.1.

1. Why is patient access a critical point in the revenue cycle process?

2. What are the comparative advantages and disadvantages of centralized, decentralized, and hybrid approaches to patient registration?

3. List three factors that can lead to failure to identify a patient's existing medical record number.

Figure 4.2. Examples of visits, encounters, and account number assignment

- A patient visits the facility for a laboratory test on Monday. The patient returns to the facility on Thursday for an x-ray. This outpatient has had two visits and two encounters. Two account numbers were assigned.
- A patient visits the facility on Monday with a script (physician orders) for a laboratory test and an x-ray, and both services are performed that day. This patient has had two visits and one encounter. One account number is assigned.
- A patient visits the facility for 12 physical therapy visits over the course of 3 weeks. The outpatient has 12 visits, one encounter, and one account number. In this example, if the therapy spans more than one calendar month, the provider may close and bill the patient account at the end of one calendar month and open a new account for the subsequent month. In this scenario, two account numbers are assigned.
- A patient comes to the emergency department (ED) on Wednesday night and is treated over the course of 10 hours. The patient is released on Thursday morning. This outpatient has had one visit and one encounter, and there will be one account number.
- A patient comes to the ED on Wednesday night and is treated over the course of 10 hours. On Thursday morning, the physician writes an order to admit the patient to the hospital. This event is now documented as an inpatient visit, with an admission date of Thursday morning and visit charges as of Wednesday: one visit, one encounter, and one account number.
- A patient comes to the ED on Wednesday and is treated and released. This is documented as one visit, one encounter, and one account. The same patient returns to the ED on Friday for the exact same problem (principal diagnosis matches to the fifth digit) and is admitted to the hospital. The second occurrence is also documented as one visit and one encounter, and it is assigned one new account number. However, the two accounts would subsequently be merged for Medicare and some other payers under the three-day payment window.
- A patient is currently an inpatient on a medical/surgical bed, and a behavioral health (BH) consultation finds that the patient needs to be admitted to the BH unit. The patient has Medicare, so the patient must be discharged from the medical/surgical unit and admitted as a new patient to the BH unit, even though the units are within the same facility with the same name and tax identification number. Readmission is required because the hospital has separate Medicare numbers for medical/surgical versus BH. Readmission would also be required if a managed-care payer has BH carved out (paid separately from the rest of the admission and possibly by a separate payer). For example, Cigna pays for medical services while Cigna Behavioral Health (CBH) pays for the BH services.

Verification of Demographics

Healthcare facilities must collect and validate patient identification at every encounter. In some cases, the registrar knows the patient. For example, a registrar may recognize fellow employees, returning therapy patients, and other frequent visitors to the facility, which makes the identification of the patient simple and highly certain. However, most patients are unknown to the registrar, making the identification process less certain. As a best practice, identification must be checked every time. In the best-case scenario, registration has an electronic system that lies on top of the hospital's registration system, and once the registrar gets to a certain field within the registration process, that field automatically launches the eligibility system to verify the patient's benefits as well as their address. The system then sends a message to let the registrar know that updated information was found.

There are two primary reasons to properly identify the patient: accuracy of the MPI and assurance of the patient's identity. The first reason was discussed earlier—accurate data is necessary to facilitate operations and identify the patient in subsequent visits. Assurance of the patient's identity, on the other hand, speaks to the facility's need to make sure that patients are who they say they are—in other words, to prevent fraudulent access.

Medical Identity Fraud and Fraud Prevention

When discussing fraud and abuse in healthcare, the first thing that may come to mind is fraudulent billing practices. However, from the facility standpoint, fraudulent access is also of concern. An individual who comes to the emergency department (ED) for treatment of a fractured bone may incur thousands of dollars of charges. Without any insurance and even with a discount, the patient may end up owing the facility a significant sum. If the patient does not present any identification at the time of treatment, the facility has no alternative but to accept and record whatever data the patient conveys. The patient could say anything and, in an emergent situation, the facility would have no choice but to provide services. The patient could, theoretically, have picked a name and address out of the phone book.

One way to facilitate the accurate collection and recording of MPI data is through the verification of the patient's demographics (identifying data) at every visit. Since these data enable the user to distinguish one patient from another, accuracy is essential. Presentation of government-issued identification containing a photograph, such as a passport or driver's license, is best. This method of identification is by no means perfect—government-issued identification can be falsified or fraudulently used by a person who looks similar to the individual issued the license or passport. However, checking government-issued identification does give the facility a measure of assurance of the patient's identity; also, state-issued identification can be used to confirm the patient's address at the time the identification was issued. If the patient presents a passport or the address has changed since the issuance of driver's license, additional documentation, such as a utility bill or credit card statement, can serve as supporting verification of the address.

Although hospitals are certainly concerned about the correct identification of patients because of the reimbursement issues, the verification of patient identities at every visit is also important because of the Red Flags Rule issued by the Federal Trade Commission (FTC). The **Red Flags Rule** requires that any organization that extends credit to a customer (in this case, a patient) must develop and implement policies and procedures to prevent, detect, report, and correct identity theft. With the rising cost of healthcare, medical identity theft has increased. **Medical identity theft** involves both the fraudulent presentation of a patient for care using someone else's identity as well as the use of an individual's identity to present fraudulent claims for reimbursement. It is the former situation against which providers must defend themselves by routinely verifying identification. The following fraudulent scenarios illustrate important reasons to verify the patient's identity and insurance coverage at every visit.

> **Example 1** Patient Smith comes to the emergency department (ED) for treatment of a broken arm. Smith is legitimately a Medicaid participant, and proper reimbursement is obtained for the treatment provided. Unknown to Smith, his uninsured cousin Brown comes to the same ED and seeks treatment for abdominal pain while claiming to be Smith. The abdominal pain is diagnosed as appendicitis, and an emergency appendectomy is performed. Brown leaves the facility, and the provider bills Medicaid for his care under Smith's name.

In this example, Smith's medical identity has been stolen. A fraud has been perpetrated against the provider and against Medicaid. Even if Smith's photo identification is on file at the facility, it will not necessarily prevent the fraud if the two men have similar facial features and other physical characteristics. Providers are required by **Emergency Medical Treatment and Active Labor Act (EMTALA)** to medically evaluate and stabilize emergent patients, and Brown's fraud is facilitated by the emergent situation. The provider has what seems to be existing demographic and financial data on file and, if Brown is alone and in pain, patient access cannot question him or anyone else, or ask for additional documentation before treatment. Nevertheless, diligence in obtaining proper identification and insurance information whenever possible will protect the provider from participating in Medicaid fraud. Further, the uninsured patient may be eligible for some other payment source and the application process can be started at point of care.

Sometimes, fraud in these situations is uncovered only when the actual patient seeks treatment of the same condition. For example, if Smith subsequently had appendicitis, Medicaid would presumably be suspicious of a claim for a second appendectomy and would deny reimbursement. Assuming the same provider is used, one hopes that the provider would realize what happened previously was fraud before it dropped a bill for Smith's legitimate care.

> **Example 2** Patient Garcia routinely receives care at Community Hospital. Over the years, she has had a broken leg and a dog bite and gave birth twice. She loses her wallet on vacation, but there wasn't much in it except her driver's license and her insurance cards, so she has the documentation replaced and never reports the loss to the police. One day, she receives an explanation of benefits (EOB) from her insurance company denying payment for an elective procedure. Shortly thereafter, she receives a bill from General Hospital for the amount due for the surgery. She calls General Hospital, demanding to see the records and claiming identity theft. General Hospital has no experience with this type of situation and refuses access to the records because she was not the patient.

In this example, Garcia erred by not reporting the loss to the police. While one does not normally think to file a police report when something is lost, the potential for identity theft is high if the lost items include specific identification, such as a driver's license. Since the patient treated under Garcia's name produced identification and insurance card that seemed valid, General Hospital would have no way of knowing that the patient was committing fraud. However, the hospital should take immediate actions following notification from Garcia of the possible fraud. Merely blocking Garcia's access to the records needed to resolve the situation is not helpful. Examples of constructive actions that might be taken include meeting with Garcia, examining supporting documentation, notifying the payer, and notifying the police. The specific actions to take should be listed in the facility's policies and procedures manual, and the bill collections process should be suspended during the investigation. A third-party payer would deny reimbursement for fraudulent billing.

> **Example 3** A registrar at Community Hospital has noticed that she can view and print patient identification documentation that has been scanned into the hospital's computer. She chooses a patient who has visited the hospital only for radiology and generates a new registration for her friend, based on the existing patient's identification, and re-scans it to the new encounter.

In this example, Community Hospital does not have sufficient security controls over patient access. If the registrar is subsequently able to delete the registration or is in collusion with an employee from patient accounting, the hospital might never notice the problem. However, effective policies and procedures to supervise, monitor, and audit registration activities should enable the provider to prevent or detect this type of identity theft.

Another way that a patient might fraudulently obtain healthcare is by using another person's identity with that person's knowledge. This type of fraud is somewhat easier with the use of documentation such as an insurance card. As long as the insurance or other coverage is valid and identification is not carefully checked, the patient is able to obtain services. Collusion between the insured patient and the individual using false identification adds to the difficulty of detection because those parties have the opportunity to identify and avoid areas of obvious risk, such as being treated for the same unique condition on two different occasions. Registrars need to examine the documentation provided and follow policies and procedures regarding verification of data. Provider management needs to ensure that policies and procedures are clear, enforceable, and properly implemented.

To avoid medical identity theft and fraud, best-practice options, such as the electronic concepts previously mentioned (the biometric palm scanner and registration eligibility and verification systems that use real-time interfaces with the payers), need to be implemented in all registration areas. However, patient access services (PAS) managers still need to conduct shadow audits, a practice where they sit with registrars to observe their processes and evaluate whether they need re-education.

Data Integrity

Registrars need to be vigilant, skeptical, and suspicious—and, at the same time, be patient-friendly, compassionate, and helpful. The goal is to obtain accurate, complete data and associate that data with the correct patient. When we consider time constraints during the registration process and the fact that patients are often stressed, it becomes clear that registration personnel must be well trained and detail oriented and also have the critical thinking skills to recognize and appropriately react to unusual situations and instances when patients resist thorough data collection.

There are multiple uses for the data collected at registration—not just billing and reimbursement. The provider has administrative uses for the data, such as market-share analysis or research. A large amount of the data collected flows through to the bill, but regulatory reporting requirements, such as state discharge data set reporting, also must be considered. For these reasons, system controls should be in place at the front end to ensure that essential fields are completed with valid, correct data. While the system should provide the flexibility of allowing a registration to be initiated in an emergent situation without a full data set, controls, such as exception reports, should be in place to alert supervisory personnel of missing data. The sooner data are collected and entered, the fewer errors will be generated at the back end. To help ensure accuracy during registration occurs, hard-stop edits should be considered in the scheduling and registration systems. A hard stop edit requires the registrar to complete the required field before moving forward. Facilities will still need to conduct audits because hard stops do not guarantee that the registrar completed the mandatory field correctly.

For example, Uniform Hospital Discharge Data Set (UHDDS) requires the collection of a core set of data elements for all discharges, including an inpatient's date of birth. Failure to capture the date of birth in the proper field prior to discharge may prevent proper grouping of the case and stop patient accounting from dropping the bill. Furthermore, any required regulatory reporting will contain this error. Fixing the error retrospectively is time consuming and may involve personnel from more than one department. Another example of a required UHDDS field is ethnicity. Once the patient has left the facility, it is difficult to accurately determine his or her ethnicity. As registrars are on the front line of data collection, the better trained and educated they are, the more likely the data they collect will be complete and accurate. Thoroughly orienting registrars to the uses and importance of the data they collect may elevate their motivation to be accurate. Incorporation of empirical data quality standards into the employee review process is helpful in enforcing accuracy.

Financial Information

In addition to collecting the patient's demographic data, patient access also captures certain financial data, such as the means of payment, the guarantor, and the reason for the visit. Although the reason for the visit is clinical data, it also initiates the financial transaction between the patient and the provider. Therefore, for our purposes here, it will be included in the financial information discussion.

Physician Orders

Although technically clinical information, the physician's scripts (orders) are the foundation for the healthcare transaction. The physician writes an order to admit, which creates an inpatient visit. Orders for diagnostic or therapeutic services direct other caregivers and technicians throughout the patient's stay. The order to discharge defines the conclusion of the episode of care. Similarly, an outpatient encounter is defined by the physician orders. If the physician writes an order for a blood test, such as a complete blood count (CBC), the facility performs the CBC and nothing else. One of the most common reasons that a bill fails is that the medical necessity for the procedure is not supported by the reason for the visit and the diagnosis. To avoid such billing problems, facilities can use an electronic option to assist with accuracy; medical necessity software is available for PAS staff to use when verifying that the diagnosis (*International Classification of Diseases, Tenth Revision, Clinical Modification [ICD-10-CM]*) code supports the procedure (Current Procedural Terminology/Healthcare Common Procedure Coding System [CPT/HCPCS]) code. For an inpatient visit, the format of the orders is standardized within the facility and reviewed by nursing as the orders are implemented. The reason for individual tests is (or should be) documented in the record—usually in the progress notes and sometimes in the order itself. However, orders for outpatient services flow directly through patient access.

Completeness

The physician order for outpatient services contains the physician identification, the orders, and the medical reason (diagnosis) for the order. Sometimes, the physician orders multiple tests, such as a CBC and an x-ray. Both tests must be listed on the order. If there are different medical reasons for the two tests, the reason for each should be specified on the order. Examples include the following:

- *Patient comes to the hospital with a script for a CBC.* The order must include the reason for the test, such as routine physical examination, anemia, or fatigue.
- *Patient comes to the hospital with a script for an abdominal ultrasound and a urinalysis.* A diagnosis of urinary tract infection, bladder stones, or abdominal pain will likely cover both procedures. If the order states that the reason for the visit is a routine physical examination or anemia, then the tests are not supported, because these are not tests that are typical for those diagnoses.
- *Patient comes to the hospital with a script for a chest x-ray and CBC prior to surgery.* The script should specifically state presurgical procedure. A script that states only cholelithiasis would not make sense, even if that were the reason for the surgery.

Accuracy

Once again, the registrar is called on to ensure that accurate data are collected. A registrar who has no background in medical terminology, no training in pathophysiology, and no understanding of ICD-10-CM coding is expected to read a script, decipher the language, ensure that the diagnoses support the order, and record the correct code that represents the diagnoses—down to the last digit. If the physician has written a complete and comprehensive script in legible handwriting and included the correct code(s), the registrar may be up to the task. One way to facilitate the communication between physician and registrar is to encourage the use of standard order forms that can either include the diagnosis codes or at least leave a space for them. To assist with this issue, hospitals are interfacing their EHR with physicians' electronic medical record (EMR) systems to be able to send scripts, review patient records, and, as needed, share other data regarding patient care for shared patients.

In a free-text script, the registrar may have trouble reading the order. Supervisory personnel can assist with this task. Sometimes, it is necessary to contact the physician's office for clarification, which can slow the registration process and impair patient satisfaction. The reason for the visit flows through to the uniform bill (UB). Therefore, clarifying the order and coding at the front end can prevent delays in billing on the back end.

Documentation

As has been previously discussed, documentation of the patient's identity must be reviewed. This documentation is either photocopied and filed or scanned into the system. Access to scanned documentation should be limited to only those individuals who need to review this documentation for legitimate business purposes. In addition to the identifying documentation, the physician order (for outpatient services) will also be retained and may be scanned or otherwise added to the patient's health record. Two additional documents that PAS is responsible for obtaining are the general consent for treatment and the notice of privacy practices. PAS is also responsible for obtaining specialized consents for behavioral health, including substance abuse and alcohol; caregiver consent; a decision-making contact; and state-level appeals notice and authorization forms. Note that caregivers and the decision-making contact might not be the patient's family members.

The form used to confirm general consent for treatment may vary depending on the type of services the patient is to receive. A simple laboratory test will not require extensive consent; an inpatient admission will require a consent that explains the general types of services the patient will receive. This general consent also contains a section in which the patient agrees to allow the provider to use the health records to obtain payment for the services and a section in which the patient agrees to pay if the third-party payer denies payment. If the patient is to have an invasive or otherwise risky procedure, an informed consent is required. A lengthy discussion of the requirements and content of such consents is outside the scope of this volume. However, figure 4.3 provides an example.

In addition to the various forms of consent, additional documentation collected at registration may include the patient's living will or medical power of attorney. The patient will also be given a statement of patient's rights, which includes information about how to file a complaint if those rights have been violated.

Finally, the Health Insurance Portability and Accountability Act (HIPAA) requires that the patient be given the provider's notice of privacy practices. Documentation of the patient's acknowledgment that the notice has been received and any questions answered must be retained. Again, this documentation can be filed or scanned. Figure 4.4 is an example.

Patient Customer Service—Front-End Transparency

An increasingly important component of the revenue cycle process is front-end transparency (the education of patients, prior to services being rendered, regarding their financial responsibilities). For example, while patients may understand the concept of co-insurance, they may not realize that they are responsible for paying $1,000 for an 80/20 split of a $5,000 covered service or might owe the full $5,000 if they have an unmet $5,000 deductible. The patient should be informed of the estimated final bill, and the provider may reasonably expect a deposit or substantial prepayment for elective services.

Patients do not always understand the relationship between their insurance plan coverage and the services being rendered. For example, a patient's physician may write a script for a blood test to verify suspected vitamin D deficiency. Many insurance plans, including Medicare, will not pay for this blood test without a corresponding diagnosis that substantiates the medical necessity of the test. In this case, osteoporosis is an example of such a diagnosis. We use this example to

Figure 4.3. Sample consent to treatment and consent to the use and disclosure of protected health information forms

University of Anystate Hospitals

CONSENT FOR TREATMENT AND DISCLOSURE
OF PROTECTED HEALTH INFORMATION
PAGE 1 OF 2

PATIENT LABEL

To the Patient (or his/her parent, guardian, or legal representative):

Before University of Anystate Hospitals and Clinics or any of its departments can provide inpatient or outpatient services to you, you will need to understand the services you are to receive, give the hospital your consent to perform those services, and agree to pay for them. You will also need to understand the ways the hospital uses the information in your health record and agree to allow the hospital to use that information.

Part I of this form covers your consent to treatment and explains other important matters related to your healthcare. Part II explains the use of your personal health information. You may ask a member of the admissions staff to read this form to you, and we encourage you to ask any questions you may have about it. When you fully understand the form's content, please sign it in the place indicated on the back of the form. Thank you very much for helping us to fulfill the hospital's responsibility to you and the rest of the community we serve.

Part I: Treatment-Related Information

Consent to the Treatment

You authorize your physician and/or other qualified medical providers to perform medical treatments and services on your behalf. You also consent to all of the hospital medical and/or diagnostic services ordered for you during your outpatient visit or inpatient stay in the hospital. This consent includes testing for infections such as hepatitis B and HIV and providing blood or body fluids for such tests in order to protect you and/or those who care for you.

Payment for Services and Insurance

You are directly responsible for paying for the services provided during your hospital visit or stay. The hospital will work directly with the third parties who provide coverage of your medical expenses, including health insurance companies, Medicare, Medicaid, Workers' Compensation, and various types of liability, accident, and disability insurance providers. By signing this form, you attest that your insurance coverage is current, valid, and effective and that you will promptly pay any required copayment amounts and unpaid deductibles. If your stay qualifies for Medicare coverage, the benefits you will receive include coverage for the physician services that were performed as part of your hospital care.

You guarantee payment to the hospital for all noncovered services and any unpaid, billed amounts not covered by insurance benefits when your insurance plan allows the hospital to bill you for any unpaid balances. You understand and accept that your physician's orders may include services not paid by insurance plans but will be provided to you by the hospital. Also, you accept that insurance plans may deny payment for what you believed were covered services, resulting in your responsibility for paying for these services. You may be billed for the professional component of any hospital services, such as the professional component for clinical laboratory tests.

Valuables

You accept full responsibility for your valuables, especially money or jewelry. The hospital does not accept any liability for your valuables. The hospital expects you will entrust any valuables to family or friends for safekeeping. Alternatively, you may deposit them in the safe that the hospital provides for that purpose. This is especially important when you are an inpatient, but this responsibility also extends to when you are an outpatient and must change into a hospital gown, remove jewelry, or undergo sedation during a medical procedure.

Special Note for Medicare or CHAMPUS Beneficiaries

You acknowledge and certify by your signature that all of the information you have provided to the hospital for Medicare or CHAMPUS benefits is correct. You also agree to allow the hospital or others who have information on your Medicare or CHAMPUS benefits claim to provide this information to Medicare or CHAMPUS or their agents in order for them to determine your eligibility for benefits. To carry out this activity, the hospital may use a copy rather than the original of this consent form. You also acknowledge that you have received a copy of the *Important Message from Medicare* or the *Important Message from CHAMPUS* form. This acknowledgement does not waive your rights for a review or make you liable for payment.

Source: AHIMA 2004.

illustrate the impact of popular media on provider and patient behavior. The patient may have read that many individuals in North America are vitamin D–deficient and wonder whether she needs to take supplements. Patient access staff need to be able to determine whether the blood test will be covered by the patient's insurance and to inform the patient if it will not. For Medicare beneficiaries, completion of an **advance beneficiary notice (ABN)** (shown in figure 4.5) will

Figure 4.4. Sample notice of health information practices

THIS NOTICE DESCRIBES HOW INFORMATION ABOUT YOU MAY BE USED AND DISCLOSED AND HOW YOU CAN GET ACCESS TO THIS INFORMATION. PLEASE REVIEW IT CAREFULLY.

Understanding Your Health Record/Information

Each time you visit a hospital, physician, or other healthcare provider, a record of your visit is made. Typically, this record contains your symptoms, examination and test results, diagnoses, treatment, and a plan for future care or treatment. This information, often referred to as your "health record" or "medical record," serves as a:

- Basis for planning your care and treatment
- Means of communication among the many health professionals who contribute to your care
- Legal document describing the care you received
- Means by which you or a third-party payer can verify that services billed actually were provided
- Tool in educating health professionals
- Source of data for medical research
- Source of information for public health officials charged with improving the health of the nation
- Source of data for facility planning and marketing
- Tool with which we can assess and continually work to improve the care we render and the outcomes we achieve

Understanding what is in your record and how your health information is used helps you to:

- Ensure its accuracy
- Better understand who, what, when, where, and why others may access your health information
- Make more informed decisions when authorizing disclosure to others

Your Health Information Rights

Although your health record is the physical property of the healthcare practitioner or facility that compiled it, the information belongs to you. You have the right to:

- Request a restriction on certain uses and disclosures of your information as provided by 45 CFR 164.522
- Obtain a paper copy of the notice of information practices upon request
- Inspect and copy your health record as provided for in 45 CFR 164.524
- Amend your health record as provided in 45 CFR 164.526
- Obtain an accounting of disclosures of your health information as provided in 45 CFR 164.528
- Request communications of your health information by alternative means or at alternative locations
- Revoke your authorization to use or disclose health information except to the extent that action has already been taken

Our Responsibilities

This organization is required to:

- Maintain the privacy of your health information
- Provide you with a notice as to our legal duties and privacy practices with respect to information we collect and maintain about you
- Abide by the terms of this notice
- Notify you if we are unable to agree to a requested restriction
- Accommodate reasonable requests you may have to communicate health information by alternative means or at alternative locations

Figure 4.4. Sample notice of health information practices (Continued)

We reserve the right to change our practices and to make the new provisions effective for all protected health information we maintain. Should our information practices change, we will mail a revised notice to the address you have supplied us.

We will not use or disclose your health information without your authorization, except as described in this notice.

For More Information or to Report a Problem

If have questions and would like additional information, you may contact the Director of Health Information Management at (444) 111-1111.

If you believe your privacy rights have been violated, you can file a complaint with the Director of Health Information Management or with the Secretary of Health and Human Services. There will be no retaliation for filing a complaint.

Examples of Disclosures for Treatment, Payment, and Health Operations

We will use your health information for treatment. For example: Information obtained by a nurse, physician, or other member of your healthcare team will be recorded in your record and used to determine the course of treatment that should work best for you. Your physician will document in your record his or her expectations of the members of your healthcare team. Members of your healthcare team will then record the actions they took and their observations. In that way, the physician will know how you are responding to treatment.

We will also provide your physician or a subsequent healthcare provider with copies of various reports that should assist him or her in treating you once you are discharged from this hospital.

We will use your health information for payment. For example: A bill may be sent to you or a third-party payer. The information on or accompanying the bill may include information that identifies you, as well as your diagnosis, procedures, and supplies used.

We will use your health information for regular health operations. For example: Members of the medical staff, the risk or quality improvement manager, or members of the quality improvement team may use information in your health record to assess the care and outcomes in your case and others like it. This information will then be used in an effort to continue improving the quality and effectiveness of the healthcare and service we provide.

Other Uses or Disclosures

Business associates: Some services in our organization are provided through contacts with business associates. Examples include physician services in the emergency department and radiology, certain laboratory tests, and a copy service we use when making copies of your health record. When these services are contracted, we may disclose your health information to our business associates so that they can perform the job we have asked them to do and bill you or your third-party payer for services rendered. So that your health information is protected, however, we require the business associate to safeguard your information appropriately.

Directory: Unless you notify us that you object, we will use your name, location in the facility, general condition, and religious affiliation for directory purposes. This information may be provided to members of the clergy and, except for religious affiliation, to other people who ask for you by name.

Notification: We may use or disclose information to notify or assist in notifying a family member, personal representative, or another person responsible for your care, location, and general condition.

Figure 4.4. Sample notice of health information practices (Continued)

Communication with family: Health professionals, using their best judgment, may disclose to a family member, other relative, close personal friend, or any other person you identify, health information relevant to that person's involvement in your care or payment related to your care.

Research: We may disclose information to researchers when their research has been approved by an institutional review board that has reviewed the research proposal and established protocols to ensure the privacy of your health information.

Funeral directors: We may disclose to funeral directors health information consistent with applicable law so they can carry out their duties.

Organ procurement organizations: Consistent with applicable law, for the purpose of tissue donation and transplant, we may disclose health information to organ procurement organizations or other entities engaged in the procurement, banking, or transplantation of organs.

Marketing: We may contact you to provide appointment reminders or information about treatment alternatives or other health-related benefits and services that may be of interest to you.

Fund-raising: We may contact you as part of a fund-raising effort.

Food and Drug Administration (FDA): We may disclose to the FDA health information relative to adverse events with respect to food, supplements, product and product defects, or postmarketing surveillance information to enable product recalls, repairs, or replacement.

Workers' compensation: We may disclose health information to the extent authorized by and to the extent necessary to comply with laws relating to workers' compensation or other similar programs established by law.

Public health: As required by law, we may disclose your health information to public health or legal authorities charged with preventing or controlling disease, injury, or disability.

Correctional institution: Should you be an inmate of a correctional institution, we may disclose to the institution or agents thereof health information necessary for your health and the health and safety of other individuals.

Law enforcement: We may disclose health information for law enforcement purposes as required by law or in response to a valid subpoena.

Federal law makes provision for your health information to be released to an appropriate health oversight agency, public health authority, or attorney, provided that a workforce member or business associate believes in good faith that we have engaged in unlawful conduct or have otherwise violated professional or clinical standards and are potentially endangering one or more patients, workers, or the public.

My signature below indicates that I have been provided with a copy of the notice of privacy practices.

_____   _____

Signature of Patient or Legal Representative   Date

If signed by legal representative, relationship to patient _____

Effective Date: _____

Distribution: Original to provider, copy to patient

Source: AHIMA 2011.

Figure 4.5. Sample advance beneficiary notice (ABN)

A. Notifier:

B. Patient Name: **C. Identification Number:**

Advance Beneficiary Notice of Noncoverage (ABN)

<u>NOTE:</u> If Medicare doesn't pay for **D.** _____ below, you may have to pay.
Medicare does not pay for everything, even some care that you or your health care provider have good reason to think you need. We expect Medicare may not pay for the **D.** _____ below.

D.	E. Reason Medicare May Not Pay:	F. Estimated Cost

WHAT YOU NEED TO DO NOW:
- Read this notice, so you can make an informed decision about your care.
- Ask us any questions that you may have after you finish reading.
- Choose an option below about whether to receive the **D.** _____ listed above.
   Note: If you choose Option 1 or 2, we may help you to use any other insurance that you might have, but Medicare cannot require us to do this.

G . OPTIONS: Check only one box. We cannot choose a box for you.

☐ **OPTION 1.** I want the **D.** _____ listed above. You may ask to be paid now, but I also want Medicare billed for an official decision on payment, which is sent to me on a Medicare Summary Notice (MSN). I understand that if Medicare doesn't pay, I am responsible for payment, but **I can appeal to Medicare** by following the directions on the MSN. If Medicare does pay, you will refund any payments I made to you, less co-pays or deductibles.

☐ **OPTION 2.** I want the **D.** _____ listed above, but do not bill Medicare. You may ask to be paid now as I am responsible for payment. **I cannot appeal if Medicare is not billed.**

☐ **OPTION 3.** I don't want the **D.** _____ listed above. I understand with this choice I am **not** responsible for payment, and **I cannot appeal to see if Medicare would pay.**

H. Additional Information:

This notice gives our opinion, not an official Medicare decision. If you have other questions on this notice or Medicare billing, call **1-800-MEDICARE** (1-800-633-4227/**TTY:**1-877-486-2048).
Signing below means that you have received and understand this notice. You also receive a copy.

I. Signature:	J. Date:

According to the Paperwork Reduction Act of 1995, no persons are required to respond to a collection of information unless it displays a valid OMB control number. The valid OMB control number for this information collection is 0938-0566. The time required to complete this information collection is estimated to average 7 minutes per response, including the time to review instructions, search existing data resources, gather the data needed, and complete and review the information collection. If you have comments concerning the accuracy of the time estimate or suggestions for improving this form, please write to: CMS, 7500 Security Boulevard, Attn: PRA Reports Clearance Officer, Baltimore, Maryland 21244-1850.

Form CMS-R-131 (03/11)   Form Approved OMB No. 0938-0566

Source: CMS 2014b.

be required prior to the service so that the hospital can bill the patient if Medicare denies payment. Similarly, facilities must comply with commercial and other payers' requirements regarding patient notification and balance billing to ensure that the provider is appropriately reimbursed for services rendered that where not authorized or are not covered. For a managed care payer, a self-pay waiver would be used (see figures 4.6 and 4.7). A self-pay waiver is similar to an ABN but refers to the insurance contract rather than Medicare.

Figure 4.6. Sample inpatient self-pay waiver

Inpatient Health Insurance Denial Form

I, _____ have been advised by _____
     (Print Name of Patient/Guardian)   (Print Name of Hospital Employee)

of the _____ department that the proposed treatment and/or
         (Print Name of Department)

continued stay is not going to be covered by my/patient's health insurance plan,

_____ – _____.
            (Please Print Managed Care Company's Name and Plan Name)

This is because (Please Check Reason for Health Insurance Denial)

_____ Hospital is a nonparticipating provider

_____ Said treatment and/or stay is considered a noncovered service

_____ Said treatment and/or stay has been deemed not medically necessary.

I am aware that, should I/patient remain in the hospital, I will be financially responsible for charges not covered by my/patient's health insurance plan effective _____ (Date).

I agree to pay [name of provider] _____

$ _____ per day for treatment with an initial deposit of $ _____.

I am aware that I have a right to appeal this denial through my/patient's health plan.

_____   _____
     Print Name of Patient/Legal Guardian   Date

_____
     Signature of Patient/Legal Guardian

Some patients may unknowingly rely on incorrect or outdated information when choosing their providers, leading to unexpected financial consequences. Patients may not realize that their plan will not pay for laboratory tests done at a hospital facility because the payer has a relationship with a stand-alone provider for such tests. In such cases, the provider must have a policy and procedure in place to support patient access personnel in either redirecting the patient to the preferred provider or obtaining payment for the service from the patient.

These are just a few examples of the types of situations that can arise when patients seek services for which they may incur a financial obligation. Providers should always be clear and helpful to patients up front regarding the potential costs to the patient and, whenever possible, provide that information in writing, obtaining a signature from the patient that the information has been received. Ultimately, the goal is that patients should never be surprised by fees after services are rendered, whether the hospital is an out-of-network facility or a participating facility.

Figure 4.7.   Sample outpatient self-pay waiver

OUTPATIENT SERVICES
HEALTH INSURANCE DENIAL FORM

The purpose of this form is to help you make an informed choice about whether or not you want to receive your hospital service at this time.

Without the necessary referral/authorization from your primary care physician / specialist, your insurance carrier, _____ will not reimburse for the non-emergent service(s) you would like to receive.

_____   _____
Name of Test(s)   Estimated Cost

Please choose from the following options.

OPTION 1

_____ Yes. I want to receive my hospital service. I understand that my insurance carrier will not pay for the services provided today and that I will be billed for this service. I agree to accept financial responsibility for these services.

OPTION 2

_____ No. I have decided not to receive my hospital service at this time.

_____   _____
Date   Signature of Patient / Legal Guardian

Note: Your health information will be kept confidential. Any information captured on this form will not be released without specific permission from you the patient / legal guardian.

Check Your Understanding 4.2.

1. Describe how to identify a patient at registration.

2. When must a patient's identity and insurance coverage be verified?

3. What is front-end transparency and why is it important?

Arrangements for Payment

With 89 percent of US citizens covered by some sort of insurance, government benefit, or other subsidy, it relatively uncommon for inpatients to self-pay (Smith and Medalia 2015). Elective procedures or therapies and uncovered services will be self-pay, meaning that patients or their guarantors pay a specific amount for each service received. But how can the provider know what is self-pay and what is covered? As mentioned in chapter 1, one of the first questions a patient is asked is, "Do you have insurance?" Except in emergent situations, the presence or absence of insurance drives the conversation with the patient about how the provider will be paid for services.

Documentation of Insurance

Patients who are insured should have documentation, usually in the form of an identification card from the insurance carrier. The card will have the name of the carrier, the plan name, the patient's name, the patient identification number, and the plan identification number. Generally, the card also includes telephone numbers for both the patient and provider to contact the carrier, the physical billing address used to submit paper claims and supporting documentation (such as medical record requests), and an electronic data interchange (EDI) number. The EDI is an electronic billing address used by patient financial services (PFS) to bill electronically, as is required by current Health Information Technology for Economical and Clinical Health Act (HITECH) regulations, which expands upon HIPAA.

To ensure that a clean and accurate insurance master exists for the registrars to choose from when selecting the payer, it is important for the revenue cycle team to be a multidisciplinary group. Generally, a subgroup from the full revenue cycle team reviews the insurance master and then brings suggestions back to the full revenue cycle committee. The subcommittee should include representatives of HIM, PFS, PAS, managed care, and information technology. The subcommittee downloads and exports the existing insurance master into a spreadsheet and then makes suggested additions or deletions to the file. PAS needs a clean insurance master to reference so managed care can more easily match each insurance master selection to the building of the payer rates in the contract management system. This helps to ensure the account flows through the contract management system and the correct contractual allowance is put on the account, which allows PFS to promptly and accurately follow up on collecting PSR.

If a patient does not have an insurance card at the time of registration, and the patient has had a prior encounter with the provider, the registrar should access a copy of the insurance card from the prior encounter for verification. It is extremely important that the existence of an insurance card or the existence of a photocopy of a card from a prior encounter is the start of the conversation about insurance, not the end. In fact, the existence of an insurance card is not proof of insurance—it is merely a reference point for the provider to begin the billing process. If the patient is covered by multiple insurance plans, all of the pertinent plans must be identified and recorded. When registering a child's information, insurance information from both parents is needed. For children, the birthday rule determines which parent's insurance is primary and which is secondary. The birthday rule is simple: The primary insurance plan for the child is that of the parent whose birth date falls first in the calendar year.

In addition to the payer, the patient must also indicate who will be the guarantor (the person responsible for paying the bill if a stated third-party payer denies payment). This responsible individual is usually the patient or his or her spouse, partner, parent, or legal guardian. The relationship between the guarantor and the patient must be specified and recorded.

Verification of Insurance

Once the patient's insurance plan has been identified, it must be verified. Verification can be done simply by calling the insurance company or by using an insurance verification service. Healthcare organizations may have an entire behind-the-scenes department for communication with payers. For example, inpatient admissions typically require a notice of admissions (NOA) to the payer and preauthorizations are generally needed for high-dollar outpatient services, such as computed tomography (CT) scans, mammography, and selected same-day procedures. The staff performing this communication function should be audited and held to the following PAS key performance indicators (KPIs):

- Number of days out cleared—This refers to how many days prior to the date of service the PAS insurance verification and authorization team has cleared the account. The goal is to send letters explaining the benefits or share some form of communication (for example, a phone call or e-mail) with the patient four weeks prior to their scheduled appointment. This may not be possible for all service lines. Clearly defined parameters should be set by service line.

- No payment denials caused by the failure of a staff member in insurance verification and authorization to verify and clear an account in advance of the patient's service, if applicable, or by the application of the wrong authorization requirements in the verification and clearance process.
- Volume productivity expectations, which will vary by hospital depending on the service line each member of the team is assigned to work. This team also does any inpatient NOA, which enters the account in the case managers' payer logs used for daily concurrent review or to manage DRG-based cases.

As we have noted previously, the fact that a patient has insurance does not mean that the specific service he or she is seeking is covered. Many services, such as elective surgery, are not covered by insurance. Further, even if the service is covered, the patient's benefits may have been exceeded in the period.

An additional complication in the verification process is the approval itself. Although the payer may conditionally approve the service, it may still deny payment for noncoverage. Noncoverage issues include subscriber nonpayment of premiums, benefit exclusions, or service exceeding policy limits.

Prior Approvals

Depending on the patient's insurance plan, prior approvals for certain services may not be required. Routine laboratory tests and x-rays, for example, may not need approval if the diagnosis on the claim indicates that the test was clearly necessary. For example, an x-ray is generally necessary when patient has a bone fracture. Many patients now have benefit plans in which the patient will incur less out-of-pocket expense for getting an x-ray at a freestanding facility rather than at a hospital. Recall the co-insurance calculation from the section on front-end transparency earlier in this chapter. Many surgeries and therapies and some diagnostic services must be approved by the patient's third-party payer before being rendered. Some third-party payers even require notification for emergency surgery, such as an emergency appendectomy. Medicare and Medicaid generally do not require preapproval for covered services; however, they will deny payment for services rendered in the absence of medical necessity. It should be noted that although managed Medicare and managed Medicaid payers tend to follow Medicare and Medicaid reimbursement rules, respectively, for processing claims, these managed payers tend to follow their commercial managed care plan rules when it comes to utilization management. Oversight from a utilization management perspective is one way that Medicare and Medicaid expect to reduce healthcare costs while ensuring that beneficiaries receive quality care. Healthcare providers therefore need take into account payer-based differences when dealing with prior approvals for managed Medicare and managed Medicaid, particularly in cases (inpatient or outpatient) where the facility would not normally need an insurance verification for a Medicare beneficiary or Medicaid recipient.

Advance Beneficiary Notices

Providers are required to give an ABN to Medicare patients. The ABN alerts the patient that if services to be provided are not covered by Medicare, the provider can seek payment from the patient. In the absence of a signed ABN, the provider may not seek payment from the patient if Medicare denies the claim. Furthermore, providers cannot ask the patient for payment for a denied claim if the ABN did not specifically list the correct codes that represent the services that Medicare considered not medically necessary.

The ABN is shown in figure 4.5 and can be downloaded from the Centers for Medicare and Medicaid (CMS) website (CMS 2014b). This form must be completed and signed by the patient (or patient's representative) before services are rendered. Failure to obtain this documentation prevents the provider from seeking payment from the patient if Medicare denies the claim.

Patient notifications apply to many providers in the Medicare fee-for-service program. Additional notices can be downloaded from the CMS website (CMS 2014c).

Financial Needs Assessment

The number of individuals without health insurance has received increasing attention in recent years. Whether citing the point-in-time US Census Bureau count or the Congressional Budget Office's estimates that reflect insurance over a period of time, the uninsured represent as much as 11 percent of the US population (Smith and Medalia 2015). That national figure, of course, does not necessarily reflect insurance coverage rates in the community in which a particular provider operates. Hospital financial counselors should screen patients for Medicaid. States that took federal money to expand the state's Medicaid program are finding that more patients qualify for Medicaid now than in the past, which reduces the amount of charity care, or free care, at hospitals. Even so, providers must expect that some percentage of their patients will be uninsured and others will be underinsured (that is, they have insurance but their coverage is very limited). Therefore, providers are in the position of having to plan for patients for whom reimbursement from a third-party payer is not available. Some patients qualify for what in some states is referred to as Plan C through Plan G Medicaid, which does not cover all services, or the patient may have a co-pay for some services. Patients who elect to purchase health insurance on the federal health insurance exchange (HIX) market and select the bronze-tiered plans will have higher out–of-pocket expenses for similar coverage as silver-tiered plans. Patients with the aforementioned Medicaid plans or lower tier HIX plans may have benefits that are not as robust as they may have thought at the time of signing up for the coverage, or they may have the coverage, but their out-of-pocket expenses will be higher. These situations may cause patients to decline health services or need payment plans to receive services.

Once again, patient access is on the front lines and must be trained to identify patients who will need payment information and financial counseling. In a busy hospital or clinic setting, it is not efficient for registrars to also do financial counseling. One anticipates that the registration process will take a matter of minutes, whereas a financial counseling session could take considerably longer. This is particularly true when the patient is willing and able to begin the application and documentation process for government assistance, such as Medicaid. Therefore, a patient access team dedicated to assisting patients with payment concerns is essential.

One has only to imagine a person seriously injured in an accident seeking care in the ED to understand why the financial assessment process is difficult. It is unlikely that the financial counseling will be effective during the patient's time in the ED. Therefore, the provider must establish follow-up procedures to ensure that patients are adequately counseled and that the provider obtains reimbursement from the appropriate source.

Self-pay

For patients with insurance, out-of-pocket expenses include any co-pay, co-insurance, or deductible amount. When coverage limits are exceeded or the patient is seeking noncovered services, even an otherwise insured patient becomes self-pay. Self-pay patients require pricing information and can be asked for deposits for non-emergent services. Per EMTALA, patients who arrive in the ED need to be triaged and deemed stabilized before staff attempt to collect insurance information or payment.

There are a number of factors to consider when a patient with no insurance or other financial assistance seeks treatment. Self-pay patients can be provided with several options, including cash payment or credit card. Depending on the facility's willingness and ability to monitor and collect over time, an installment payment plan is also an option. For elective procedures and tests, it is advisable to obtain payment in advance. Policies and procedures must be in place and enforced to ensure control over cash collections and the posting and monitoring of credit-based arrangements. Chapter 7 discusses in detail collection alternatives and discounts for self-pay at the point of service.

Occasionally, arrangements must be made for patients whose services are being covered by alternative means, such as patients participating in certain research studies and patients who have arranged for elective procedures through their surgeon or another provider. For example, an inpatient from Hospital A is transported to Hospital B for a cardiac catheterization during the inpatient stay and is then returned to Hospital A following the procedure. Typically, Hospital A would bill the third-party payer for the inpatient stay and all of the services received by the patient. Hospital B would bill Hospital A for the cardiac catheterization. However, depending upon how Hospital A and Hospital B negotiate their payer contracts, Hospital A could get an authorization from the payer for the patient to go to Hospital B because the patient needs services Hospital A is not licensed to provide. Hospital B would then bill out for the outpatient cardiac catheterization. This is contingent upon the payer; Medicare and Medicaid have very different regulations regarding this type of scenario.

Government Payers

Identification of third-party payers includes government payers, such as Medicare and Medicaid. Patients who are eligible for government coverage are not always enrolled. Patients who are enrolled are not always covered for the services they are seeking. Some patients, for example, may have exhausted their Medicare Part A coverage and have only Part B remaining. The sooner that coverage and eligibility details are verified, the better able the provider is to ensure that billing is done correctly.

As mentioned, the provider can assist patients to apply for government programs, such as Medicaid. Prior to application, the patient will be listed as self-pay. When the patient subsequently is approved for Medicaid, the provider can be changed. Some hospitals have pending Medicaid and pending charity-care options in their insurance master. These options are used so that hospital's financial counselor or the third-party vendor can easily identify the accounts that will be converted to Medicaid or charity care, if approved. In other cases, the patient has already been accepted into the Medicaid or Medicare program, but he or she does not have documentation at the time of registration. There are a number of issues that can arise in such situations. For example, certification of days for utilization is an important step in the billing process for Medicaid and Medicare. For a self-pay patient, that step would not have been taken. Therefore, a delayed posting of Medicaid or Medicare as a payer (either primary or secondary) would further delay billing until that step is completed. Allowing PAS staff access to the Medicare and Medicaid portals allows them to look up patients to verify eligibility and benefits. Verification should be done each time the patient comes in for services to determine whether Medicare Part A benefits have been exhausted; check whether the patient still needs to pay any remaining co-insurance or deductible amounts; confirm that patient has not selected or chosen to have a managed Medicare or managed Medicaid plan; and verify general eligibility.

Other Data Collection Issues

One of the primary tenets of good data collection is to collect all of the data that are needed, but not more than are needed. Individual registrars cannot be expected to know the importance of the data they collect and record unless they are trained properly. One important component of registrar training is to orient them to the uses of registration data and the impact their errors have on other departments as well as the hospital itself. A necessary digit left off an ICD-10-CM diagnosis code at registration can cause the bill to fail until the code is corrected. When registrars are expected to enter diagnosis codes provided by physicians and other clinical personnel, such as for outpatient radiology testing, facilities should develop and implement internal controls to ensure that the codes are complete and correct. A medical necessity system or module within the patient access system could assist with reducing coding errors at registration.

To understand the potential magnitude of a diagnosis coding error, assume that one registrar has the code N39 stuck in her head. She believes it means urinary tract infection (UTI) and enters the three digits whenever the patient has a script for a urinalysis to rule out UTI. However, the correct code is N39.0. If the registrar makes this error once a day for 200 days in the year and the charge for urinalysis is $50, this one registrar has held up $10,000 in laboratory charges. Furthermore, when the accounts fail to bill due to the invalid code, patient accounting must review them. It takes a patient accounting biller three minutes to correct this error each time it occurs, because the biller must review the script, correct the data entry, and rebill the account. Three minutes multiplied by 200 occurrences equals 600 minutes (10 hours) of the patient accounting biller's time. If the facility pays the biller $15 an hour, correcting this one repeat error costs the provider $150 of biller time. Assume the provider actually receives reimbursement of 40 percent of its charges (in this case, $4,000), and the aggregate cost of these tests is $3,850, which yields net revenue of $150 from the cases coded by the registrar. In this scenario, the provider has just spent all of its marginal earnings correcting a mistake that should never have been made. Thus, front-end validity edits are an important component of the registration process.

Data Quality Control

Because there is a high potential for human error in the data collection process at registration, computer-based validation edits are a very important preventive control. These edits can be as simple as alerting the registrar that an invalid entry has been keyed, such as a date that does not exist (for example, February 30), a birth date in the mid-1800s, or an invalid diagnosis code. Examples of other computer-based edit and alert functions include, but are not limited to, the following:

- Searching the MPI to alert the registrar that the current patient may have a previous medical record number that the registrar has not selected for this encounter
- Preventing the registrar from proceeding with the registration until certain critical fields are completed
- Reminding the registrar to collect a deposit from a self-pay patient, a co-pay, or a co-insurance fee

Quality assurance is a must in the registration data collection process. Routine, systematic audits of every registrar's work are essential. As has been illustrated earlier in this chapter, the provider cannot afford to employ registrars who do not have an extremely high accuracy rate. In this function, a performance improvement target goal for data collection should be 100 percent accuracy.

As we have spent considerable space discussing patient demographics, it should be clear that patient identification is a critical component of managing the revenue cycle as well as delivering patient care. The Office of the National Coordinator for Health Information Technology (ONCHIT) has published the Safety Assurance Factors for EHR Resilience (SAFER) Guide to delineate best practices with respect to patient identification in the EHR and provide users with self-assessments to identify potential problem areas (ONC 2014). Here are the 14 elements of best practice in the self-assessment:

1. An enterprise-wide master patient index that includes patients' demographic information and medical record number(s) from different parts of the same organization is used to identify patients before importing data.
2. Clinicians can select patient records from electronically generated lists based on specific criteria (e.g., user, location, time, service).

3. Information required to accurately identify the patient is clearly displayed on all computer screens, wristbands, and printouts.
4. Patient names on adjacent lines in the EHR display are visually distinct.
5. Medical record numbers incorporate a "check digit" to help prevent data entry errors.
6. Users are warned when they attempt to create a new record for a patient (or look up a patient) whose first and last name are the same as another patient.
7. Patients are registered using a centralized, common database using standardized procedures.
8. The user interfaces of the training, test, and read-only backup versions of the EHR are clearly different from the production ("live") version to prevent inadvertent entry or review of patient information in the wrong system.
9. The organization has a process to assign a "temporary" unique patient ID (which is later merged into a permanent ID) in the event that either the patient registration system is unavailable or the patient is not able to provide the required information.
10. Patient identity is verified at key points or transitions in the care process (e.g., rooming patient, vital sign recording, order entry, medication administration, and check out).
11. The EHR limits the number of patient records that can be displayed on the same computer at the same time to one, unless all subsequent patient records are opened as "Read Only" and are clearly differentiated to the user.
12. Patients who are deceased are clearly identified as such.
13. The use of test patients in the production (i.e., "live") environment is carefully monitored. When they do exist, they have unambiguously assigned "test" names (e.g., including numbers or multiple ZZ's) and are clearly identifiable as test patients (e.g., different background color for patient header).
14. The organization regularly monitors their patient database for patient identification errors. (ONC 2014)

Note that the SAFER guidelines do not all speak specifically to patient access data collection; however, items 5, 6, 7, and 9 directly address practices in patient access. Item 5 references a *check digit,* which is a digit added to an assigned number that results in a specified result when all digits are entered correctly. There are numerous algorithms to calculate a check digit. The point is to perform a calculation with the digits that results in a single correct answer. That single correct answer is then appended to the assigned number. When the assigned number plus check digit is typed into the system, the calculation is performed to determine whether the check digit is valid. If it is not, the system issues an alert that requires the user to correct the data entry. This validation check helps to prevent data-entry errors on a known health record number.

As item 6 indicates, users should be automatically warned whenever they attempt to create a new record for a patient (or look up a patient) whose first and last name are the same as another patient. Although this alert may seem redundant, it does help prevent both the creation of duplicate health records as well as inadvertent access to the wrong patient's record.

The use of a centralized, common database for patient registration (item 7) as well as standardized procedures is critical to maintaining a clean MPI. System alerts and prompts when duplication is potentially occurring help prevent duplicate entries.

Finally, the ability to assign a temporary identification number (item 9) acknowledges the fact that no electronic system is entirely free of downtime, a period of time in which the system is inaccessible due to planned activities such as updates or unplanned activities such as system failure. The process for assigning such numbers depends on the system but generally involves maintaining a set of medical record numbers and account numbers that are preregistered as "downtime" numbers that can then be assigned when the system is inaccessible. When the system comes back up, the patient documentation associated with the downtime can either be merged with the patient's existing records or, in the case of new patient, permanently assigned to that patient.

Compliance

Patient access personnel must comply with a variety of policies and procedures, including the FTC's Red Flags Rule, HIPAA privacy and security regulations, and the provider's internal policies and procedures. As with all provider personnel, the annual review of corporate compliance and HIPAA is essential in patient access.

For revenue cycle purposes, registrars should also comply with coding guidelines and other regulatory data-collection guidelines. According to the Office of Inspector General compliance plan, correct coding is critical to compliance (OIG 1998). The National Correct Coding Initiative further supports this position. Failure to collect and record the correct diagnosis code at registration not only contributes to delayed billing and denied claims but also erodes the provider's compliance position with respect to correct coding. For this reason, policies and procedures must be in place to ensure that registrars have the support they need to select and record the correct reason for visit or admitting diagnosis codes. Although HIM department coders will review and validate these codes in cases that they code for discharge diagnosis (see chapter 6), the HIM department does not see the coding for many outpatient areas such as laboratories and radiology. Therefore, these codes flow directly into billing and may drop to the UB without human intervention. Thus, the accuracy of the registrar's coding in many cases directly affects the bill.

Training

Ideally, patient access registrars are highly trained specialists who meet specific academic and training requirements. In fact, the National Association of Healthcare Access Management (NAHAM) has developed a set of standards for baseline education, credentialing, and continuing education for its members. Medical terminology, coding, and an overview of the revenue cycle are included in the baseline for certification. That education outline is included in the online materials that accompany this book.

In the absence of other training, the provider should ensure that registrars are well grounded in medical terminology, diagnosis coding for medical necessity, customer service, and HIPAA requirements as they pertain to the patient access function. Orientation to the position should include an overview of the charge collection (see chapter 5), chart completion, and billing functions. Finally, registrars should become experts at using the computer systems that facilitate data collection. NAHAM offers certifications exams for patient access professionals. The competency areas are included in the online materials that accompany this text (NAHAM 2015). It may occur to the HIM-trained reader that patient access is not only a potential entry-level opportunity for health information students but also a possible career path for credentialed professionals. HIM training is an acceptable foundation for NAHAM examinations for the Certified Healthcare Access Manager (CHAM) and Certified Healthcare Access Associate (CHAA).

Confidentiality

Patient access personnel are on the front lines of compliance with HIPAA privacy and security rules. They often see neighbors, friends, and coworkers as patients, and people who are well known to the general public, such as celebrities, may come to a facility for care.

While maintenance of confidentiality is not one's first thought when considering the revenue cycle, breach of confidentiality exposes the provider to the risk of legal action as well as penalties from regulatory bodies, such as the Office of Civil Rights, which enforces HIPAA. Therefore, strict application of policies and procedures regarding patient privacy and confidentiality is essential.

Special Considerations for Specific Practice Settings

For the most part, the registration process is similar across settings. Registrars collect demographic and financial data, usually enter those data into a computer system, and obtain scripts, orders, and consents for treatment as well as other documentation, such as ABNs. In facilities with multiple practice settings, registrars must also accurately record the patient's diagnostic or treatment location. For example, an ED patient is registered as an ambulatory patient. If the patient is subsequently admitted, patient access must change the patient's status to inpatient and indicate that the patient is occupying a bed. Failure to register the patient properly in this regard will result in an incorrect bill type and a failed bill. (See chapter 5 for a discussion of charges and bill types.)

Inpatient Settings

In an inpatient setting, registrars collect the foundation data for the UHDDS, which can be viewed in the recommendations for core health data elements on the NCVHS website (NCVHS 1996). Note that of the 21 data items, almost half are collected at registration: items 01–05, 07–09, and 19. This data set populates the uniform bill (discussed in detail in chapter 5).

Outpatient Settings

In an outpatient setting, registrars collect the foundation data for the Uniform Ambulatory Care Data Set (UACDS). More than half of the data elements (1–9) are collected at registration (NCVHS 1996). This data set also populates the uniform bill (discussed in detail in chapter 5).

Physician Practices

Many physician practices do not do their own billing, which is laborious. They contract a billing service to perform this function. Therefore, the data needed to populate a bill must be captured in a manner appropriate for that relationship. Physician practices often capture the bulk of their visit data on a superbill or encounter form (which is discussed in more detail in chapter 5). As physician offices move to an EHR environment, the data captured on a superbill can automatically populate an automated billing system. Provided that the physician is properly trained in the use of the clinical system, this automation provides a clear match between the services rendered and the claim.

Check Your Understanding 4.3.

1. When is prior approval for services needed?

2. What is an advance beneficiary notice?

3. List three errors that can be prevented with automated front-end validity edits.

References

42 CFR 489.24: Special responsibilities of Medicare hospitals in emergency cases. 2004.

American Health Information Management Association (AHIMA). 2011. Notice of Privacy Practices (Updated). Appendix A: Sample Notice of Privacy Practices. http://library.ahima.org/xpedio/groups /public/documents/ahima/bok1_048807.hcsp?dDocName=bok1_048807.

Centers for Medicare and Medicaid Services (CMS). 2014a. Medicare Acute Inpatient PPS Three Day Payment Window. http://www.cms.gov/Medicare/Medicare-Fee-for-Service-Payment/AcuteInpatientPPS/Three_Day _Payment_Window.html.

Centers for Medicare and Medicaid Services. 2014b. Advance Beneficiary Notice (ABN). http://www.cms .gov/Medicare/Medicare-General-Information/BNI/ABN.html.

Centers for Medicare and Medicaid Services. 2014c. Beneficiary Notices Initiative (BNI). http://www.cms .hhs.gov/BNI.

National Association of Healthcare Access Management (NAHAM). 2015. NAHAM Examination for Certified Healthcare Access Manager (CHAM) and Certified Healthcare Access Associate (CHAA) Candidate

Guide. http://c.ymcdn.com/sites/www.naham.org/resource/resmgr/certification/naham_candidate_guide _to_cer.pdf.

National Committee on Vital and Health Statistics (NCVHS). 1996. Preliminary Recommendations for Core Health Data Elements. http://www.cdc.gov/nchs/data/ncvhs/nchvs94.pdf.

New Jersey Administrative Code (NJAC). 2012 (June). Hospital Licensing Standards, NJAC. 8:43G-15.1,b. http://www.njha.com/media/302738/2012-June-NJ-Hospital-Licensing-Standards-2.pdf.

Office of Inspector General (OIG). 1998. Publication of the OIG Compliance Program for Hospitals. *Federal Register* 63(35).

Office of the National Coordinator for Health Information Technology (ONC). 2014. SAFER Self Assessment Guides. https://www.healthit.gov/sites/default/files/safer/pdfs/safer_patientidentification_sg006_form.pdf.

Smith, J.C. and C. Medalia. 2015. Health Insurance Coverage in the United States: 2014. US Census Bureau. http://www.census.gov/content/dam/Census/library/publications/2015/demo/p60-253.pdf.

Documentation and Charge Capture

Learning Objectives

- Examine the differences between inpatient and outpatient accounts.
- Illustrate the impact of a documentation improvement program on revenue cycle management.
- Compare documentation and charges.
- Create an effective chargemaster maintenance process.
- Develop internal controls to ensure reconciliation of orders and monitoring of charges.

Key Terms

- Accounts
- Charge description master
- Chargemaster
- Clinical documentation improvement
- Corrective controls
- Detective controls
- Level charge
- Preventive controls

If it's not documented, it didn't happen. This adage applies to many industries and situations. In healthcare, it applies specifically to the interaction between the patient and the caregivers. In addition to providing a legal record of this interaction, documentation also supports the charges. A physician who visits an inpatient in the hospital every day must document each day's interaction or lose the right to bill for that visit. Similarly, the hospital must ensure that appropriate documentation exists for every service rendered for the same reason.

Accounts

As explained in chapter 4, a medical record number is assigned to the patient during the registration process. The purpose of the medical record number is to facilitate identification of the patient as unique from other patients. Functionally, it also allows the system to capture and store demographic data about the patient separate and apart from the individual encounter data. For users of the individual encounter data, the medical record number also allows the user to identify all encounters under one record number. Individual encounter data are collected in separate accounts. So, a patient should have only one medical record number but may have many account numbers. The medical record number attaches to the demographic data and the account number attaches to the clinical and financial data associated with the specific encounter. For postdischarge storage and retrieval purposes, individual accounts are usually maintained in separate folders and filed by medical record number. Similarly, in an electronic health record (EHR) environment, patient data can be referenced by medical record number and by account number. When reviewing electronic patient data, it is important to ensure that one is referencing the correct time period and service because some data, such as laboratory values, may display even though is the data are associated with a different account number. It is also important to remember that the way data is displayed on an electronic dashboard does not necessarily reflect how the data were collected. Patient account data, laboratory data, nursing notes, and medication orders may be configured to display on the same screen even though they are collected at different times and by different individuals and are actually stored in separate tables in the EHR system. Therefore, when querying for data, be sure to ask for the exact data by name, not by the screen on which you have seen the data displayed.

Account documentation supports the claim for the individual encounter. Therefore, the documentation for each account must stand on its own merits and must match the charges in the claim. All diagnostic and therapeutic data should be collected in a manner that tracks directly to the claim.

Types of Accounts

There are two types of patients: inpatient and outpatient. The fundamental difference between the two types of patients is the physician's order to admit. A physician orders an inpatient admission when the patient's condition requires at least an overnight stay and 24-hour nursing care.

Inpatient length of stay is measured in days, counting the day of admission and not counting the day of discharge. In addition to 24-hour nursing care, inpatients also receive room and board and are located in an area of the hospital specifically designed to accommodate such services. Recent changes in Medicare payment rules require that physicians attest to the need for the patient to stay two nights. Called the two-midnight rule, this change seeks to establish a clearer demarcation between inpatient and outpatient services (particularly as outpatient status relates to the Centers for Medicare and Medicaid Services [CMS] observation services rule). For fiscal year 2016, CMS further clarified that stays briefer than two days would be reviewed on a case-by-case basis and emphasized that the physician's judgment and documentation of medical necessity are what support inpatient admission (CMS 2015a). It is important to keep abreast of changes in this rule, which has a significant impact on claim denials, and therefore reimbursement, to ensure that documentation supports the medical necessity of an inpatient admission.

To a hospital, an outpatient is any patient who has not been admitted. More specifically, outpatients are associated with certain departments, such as clinic, laboratory, radiology, same-day surgery, and emergency. Outpatient services are measured by encounters or visits. (Refer to chapter 4 for a discussion of the distinction between encounters and visits.) A single encounter may contain several visits or services. For example, an outpatient encounter may include a visit to the laboratory for blood tests and a visit on the same day to radiology for an x-ray. This encounter would be captured in one account. If those visits took place on different days, the patient would be registered for two different accounts because one account is typically used only for outpatient services that take place on the same day. There are a number of exceptions to this general rule. Emergency department (ED) encounters, for example, may cross over from one day to the next, resulting in different dates for the beginning and end of service. This is not a problem because the period represents one episode of service. Recurring encounters, such as those for physical therapy or chemotherapy, may be captured in one account and billed periodically, usually monthly, until the patient is discharged from that service. It is important to keep charges for these recurring encounters separate from other encounters that may occur during the same time period. For example, a laboratory visit would not be included in an unrelated recurring account for physical therapy services.

Another type of outpatient is the observation patient. Observation patients are technically outpatients because they have not been admitted to inpatient status. However, they receive room, board, and continuous nursing care. Some hospitals maintain a distinct observation unit or specific observation beds. Other hospitals integrate the observation patients with the inpatients. This latter arrangement can be confusing for patients, who sometimes assume that they are inpatients because they are on a nursing unit. As mentioned earlier in this chapter, one of the reasons for the CMS two-midnight rule is to make a clearer distinction between inpatient and observation status. The important distinction is that the physician order for outpatients in nursing units will state *observation status*. One way to ensure correct patient status is to include patient status on a physician order form for initial orders. Another distinction is that the length of stay of an observation patient is measured in hours. Regardless of the duration of the observation, the encounter is represented by one account.

The status of a patient's stay does not always remain the same type. Sometimes, the status changes from outpatient to inpatient or vice-versa. The change might occur as medical necessity dictates or due to clerical error. For example, a patient encounter may start in the ED, during which the physician decides to order an inpatient admission. This is not a new encounter. In this case, the patient type changes from outpatient to inpatient, and certain outpatient accounts would need to be included in the inpatient bill if they occur within the three-day payment window (CMS 2014a). Accurate billing when a change in patient type has occurred is most easily accomplished by combining the accounts. On the other hand, if the physician orders "observation status" but the registrar enters the patient as an inpatient, this clerical error must be corrected to bill the account correctly. In either event, the change in patient status has an effect on data collection; for example, room-and-board charges must be documented for an inpatient stay.

Impact on Data Collection

Correct classification of the patient at registration and throughout the encounter is critical for data collection (see chapter 4). An ED outpatient account is expected to contain an evaluation and management (E/M) charge for emergency services (called a **level charge**) that expresses the level of complexity and intensity of services provided and corresponds to the Common Procedural Terminology (CPT) code that describes that level of service. If the patient is subsequently admitted to inpatient status, then daily room-and-board charges will be added to the account. Delay in changing the patient's status from outpatient to inpatient may result in missed charges. For example, a patient arrives in the ED at noon. At 9 p.m., the physician writes the order for the patient to be admitted as an inpatient. If the patient's status is not changed until the next morning, the account will miss the overnight posting of room charges for the first day of service. If not corrected, the bill will fail because the room charges do not match the length of stay.

Another key factor affected by the patient type is the preauthorization for services. Some payers require prior or concurrent authorization for services before the facility can bill for those services. An authorization for a computed tomography (CT) scan of the brain would not necessarily encompass an immediately subsequent cerebral endarterectomy and an inpatient stay. Therefore, solid lines of communication are necessary between the clinical departments and patient access so that changes in patient type are properly recorded and, if necessary, authorized by the payer.

Complete Documentation

The extent to which various providers and caregivers must document healthcare services is the subject of state facility licensure regulations as well as Joint Commission, payer, and facility guidelines. Over and above the regulatory and institutional requirements are the professional standards that caregivers must follow within their own disciplines. For revenue cycle purposes, the documentation must reflect the medical necessity (the diagnostic or therapeutic rationale) for the charges, and the charges should include what is documented. For example, the need for a transfusion is reflected in documentation of blood loss anemia; the charges will include the diagnostic blood test, the blood type and cross-match, and the transfusion charge itself. When there is a discrepancy between charges and documentation, the payer may deny the bill.

Impact of Hybrid Records

Documentation to support the claim must be accessible and transmittable in a format acceptable to the payer. Payers frequently request copies of health records to review the documentation. If the payer wants a complete health record, all components must be accessible and printable for the payer (or scanned for electronic transmission). In a fully electronic environment, the specific documentation requested can be exported in a usable format—either printed in a report format for mailing, converted to an electronic document (such as a PDF file), or transmitted electronically through an interface such as HL7. In a fully paper environment, specific pages of the record can be photocopied. A true hybrid record, which has both electronic and paper components, increases the difficulty of releasing information. To ensure accurate and complete documentation, clinicians must be trained to document services in the correct place. For example, if history and physical reports are to be dictated and signed electronically, then all physicians should do so consistently. Having similar reports in both hard-copy and electronic formats is confusing.

In addition to release-of-information concerns, the documentation requirements for clinical personnel must be clear from charting to authentication.

Clinical Documentation Improvement

Clinical documentation improvement is a process an organization undertakes to improve clinical specificity and documentation so that clinical documentation is clear for reimbursement purposes. Clinicians are taught to document their investigation of a patient complaint—the clinician's point of view. The clinician's point of view, however, is not always consistent with the classification system used to convert the clinical data to classification format. Anemia is an example of this issue. As illustrated in table 5.1, the *International Classification of Diseases, Tenth Revision, Clinical Modification (ICD-10-CM)* makes more than two dozen classifications for anemia available to the coder in health information management (HIM); however, the physician documentation often consists of only one word, *anemia*.

Further complicating the communication between physician and coder is the implementation of Medicare severity diagnosis-related groups (MS-DRGs) for inpatient prospective payment system (IPPS). This severity-adjusted methodology has increased the need for specificity and detail in physician documentation that clinicians are not necessarily trained to provide. For example, traditionally, physicians document "congestive heart failure." However, severity-adjusted MS-DRGs increase the weight of certain visits only in the presence of additional clarification. The specification of diastolic or systolic congestive heart failure is a comorbidity/complication (CC) in many cases. The further specification of *acute* or *acute on chronic* congestive heart failure is a major comorbidity/complication (MCC) in many cases. The addition of a CC or MCC can bump the case into a higher weighted MS-DRG, which increases the reimbursement. In addition to the reimbursement implications, increased specificity also facilitates care management and epidemiological studies.

Analysis

Audits, claims denials, and recurring edits are good places to start when identifying areas that need improvement. In *Clinical Documentation Improvement: Achieving Excellence*, facilities are advised to use comparative data to benchmark their data and to use coded data to evaluate current performance as well as ongoing CDI program success (Hess 2014, 75-101). For example, assuming comparative data are available, CDI programs can compare staffing against discharges, percentage

Table 5.1. Selected coding classifications for anemia

ICD-10-CM Code	Code Description
D50.0	Iron deficiency anemia secondary to blood loss (chronic)
D50.1	Sideropenic dysphagia
D50.8	Other iron deficiency anemias
D50.9	Iron deficiency anemia, unspecified
D51.0	Vitamin B12 deficiency anemia due to intrinsic factor deficiency
D51.1	Vitamin B12 deficiency anemia due to selective vitamin B12 malabsorption with proteinuria
D51.2	Transcobalamin II deficiency
D51.3	Other dietary vitamin B12 deficiency anemia
D51.8	Other vitamin B12 deficiency anemias
D51.9	Vitamin B12 deficiency anemia, unspecified
D52.0	Dietary folate deficiency anemia
D52.1	Drug-induced folate deficiency anemia
D52.8	Other folate deficiency anemias
D52.9	Folate deficiency anemia, unspecified
D53.0	Protein deficiency anemia
D53.1	Other megaloblastic anemias, not elsewhere classified
D53.2	Scorbutic anemia
D53.8	Other specified nutritional anemias
D53.9	Nutritional anemia, unspecified
D55.0	Anemia due to glucose-6-phosphate dehydrogenase [G6PD] deficiency
D55.1	Anemia due to other disorders of glutathione metabolism
D55.2	Anemia due to disorders of glycolytic enzymes
D55.3	Anemia due to disorders of nucleotide metabolism
D55.8	Other anemias due to enzyme disorders
D55.9	Anemia due to enzyme disorder, unspecified
D64.0	Anemia, unspecified (If further documentation is not provided, the coder must use this term, which may not satisfy medical necessity for some services.)

of cases reviewed on a timely basis, percentage of cases for which documentation clarifications were recommended, and percentage of documentation clarifications that were affected prior to discharge. These comparisons are also useful longitudinally within the program to set goals and demonstrate performance improvement. While documentation clarification certainly supports medical necessity and coding specificity, such clarification may also result in diagnosis-related group (DRG) changes. Therefore, tracking the percentage of reviewed cases that resulted in a change in DRG can be benchmarked, and the associated change in expected revenue is a tangible result that can help demonstrate the impact of the program on the revenue cycle.

Education

Although the ostensible purpose of a CDI program is to improve physician documentation, it is in reality a method to improve *communication*, which is the primary purpose of documentation. By documenting, the physician is communicating with nurses for clinical care and other physicians in the course of diagnosing and planning treatment for the patient. Documentation improvement facilitates those relationships as well as communication with case management, coders, and payers. The more clearly and succinctly the physician communicates, the better able these parties are to respond appropriately.

Although a complete discussion of CDI programs is beyond the scope of this text, it should be noted that a robust query process is extremely helpful in postdischarge communication between physicians and coders. See chapter 6 for a detailed discussion of the query process.

Tracking

To measure the success of a CDI program, one must evaluate it in the context of the goals of the program. At a minimum, one would expect use of a CDI program to improve coding accuracy and reduce claims denials for medical necessity. Of course, administration would tend to expect an increase in case-mix index (CMI), because that results in increased reimbursement (at least for Medicare cases). Table 5.2 lists some potential goals of a CDI program and possible measures of success. Any measure of success to be tracked should be identified and recorded prior to implementation of the program to ensure accurate evaluation of the program.

Table 5.2. CDI program goals and measures of success

Goal	Measures	Explanation
Improved communication between physicians and coders	Number of postdischarge queries Days in query	Once the program is running smoothly, the number of queries necessary postdischarge should decline. Similarly, as physicians buy into the concepts, their response times to queries should also improve.
Reduced postdischarge coding time	Days in discharged, no final bill (DNFB) DNFB dollars	Because the chart is being reviewed concurrently, and queries are addressed concurrently, the length of time between discharge and query resolution should shorten. Further, the dollars associated with those queries will be billed sooner, reducing overall DNFB.
Reduced denials for medical necessity	Number of denials Percentage of overturned denials Audit rate	As physicians become more attuned to the specific documentation requirements, their specificity may yield the added benefit of reducing denials. Certainly, the number of denials that are overturned on appeal will be increased if physicians significantly improve documentation. Further, the rate at which payers audit facility records may decline as such audits yield fewer benefits to the payer.

Check Your Understanding 5.1.

1. Distinguish between inpatient and outpatient accounts.

2. Why is a CDI program necessary?

3. What are the key components of a CDI program?

Charges

The services that patients receive must be tracked. Departments need to know how many procedures were performed, supplies were used, and patients were seen. Patient accounting needs to know how much to bill the patient or other payer. The payer wants to know whether the services rendered match what was authorized or otherwise payable. Consequently, a detailed listing of services and charges must be accumulated in the account. For a detailed discussion of how charges become revenue and why this is important, see chapter 2.

The anatomy of a charge consists of the date of service, the responsible department, a description of the service, and the volume and price for the service. An example is shown in table 5.3.

In this ED example, the charge for the complete blood count (CBC) with differential laboratory test was entered on the date of service, the level charge of ED visit, Level 3 was entered the next day, and the radiology charge was entered four days later (a late charge).

Charge Description Master

Similar to a grocery store, which keeps detailed records of every possible item to be sold so that purchases can be scanned at checkout, a provider must also maintain a list of every possible charge that could go into an account. This master list is called the chargemaster or charge description master (CDM). The CDM is a database of all the supplies and services provided to patients and the corresponding charges for those items. The key field in the database is the charge code—the unique identifier for each charge. Other fields in the CDM provide additional detail.

The CDM enables the facility to capture and record patient charges efficiently as they are incurred. In addition to capturing charges for billing, the CDM can provide data for budgeting by providing statistics on volume for both individual departments as well as services. Charges can also be compared to actual costs of providing services to determine the profitability of given services and departments. An example of a charge description master is shown in table 5.4. The structure and maintenance of the CDM depends on the system used, but the basic components are similar. Table 5.5 explains the individual fields in the sample CDM as well as some fields that are not shown in the CDM example in table 5.4.

Various payers may have different requirements regarding payments of specific charges in the CDM database—for example, certain payers may deem selected items in the CDM to be non-payable. Also, some payers recognize certain Healthcare Common Procedure Coding System (HCPCS) codes as opposed to CPT codes, and this specification needs to be noted by payer in the CDM to bill payers correctly. The specific charge requirements for inpatient charges versus outpatient charges may also differ.

Some charges inherently go together, such as the those for the injection of a vaccine. There is one code for the vaccine itself and another for the injection. The facility may choose to set up one code that "explodes" into two charges, a convention that is more administratively efficient for staff who are responsible for recording all charges. In other words, the user enters one code and

Table 5.3. Anatomy of a charge for an ED visit, 9 a.m.–3 p.m. on 10/12/2015

Date of Service	Date Posted	Revenue Code	CPT/HCPCS Code	Description	Modifier(s)	Volume	Price
10/12/2015	10/12/2015	305	85004	CBC with differential		1	$ 165
10/12/2015	10/12/2015	309	36415	Phlebotomy		1	$ 50
10/12/2015	10/13/2015	450	99283	ED visit, Level 3	25	1	$2,400
10/12/2015	10/16/2015	324	71010	Chest x-ray		1	$ 300

CPT codes © American Medical Association 2015. All rights reserved.

Table 5.4. Sample CDM

Charge Code	Item Description	CPT/HCPCS Code				G/L Key	Activity Date
		INS Code A	Rev Code A	INS Code B	Rev Code B		
52526944	Filgrastim inj 300mcg/1ml (IV)		250	J1440	636	3	8/1/2006
52511730	Calcitonin inj 400units/2ml		250	J0630	636	3	7/26/2015
52528239	Cytomegalovirus imm glob 2.5gm		250	J0850	636	3	6/25/2015
54600663	Exercise oximetry evaluation	94761	460	94761	460	3	5/24/2015
54600325	Flutter valve training sec clr	94667	460	94667	460	3	4/25/2015
56208903	Bentson guidewire 035/145		272	C1769	621	2	7/3/2015
56208846	Rosen guidewire 035/145/1.5		272	C1769	621	2	8/14/2014
54001284	Echo encephalogram	76506	402	76506	402	3	7/21/2015
53200168	Sinuses; paranasal. complt	70220	320	70220	320	3	7/13/2015
53002010	Bilirubin total	82247	301	82247	301	3	8/8/2015
57100117	Recovery phase 0.5 hr		710		710	3	3/12/2015
56221609	Wallstent iliac 12mm/90mm		272	C1876	278	2	7/8/2015
59200071	US; duplex. abdm/pelvc, lmtd	93976	921	93976	921	3	5/16/2015
52502341	Varicella vaccine inj 0.5ml		250	90716	636	3	8/1/2015
52502390	Pneumococcal vaccine 0.5ml		250	90732	636	3	7/26/2015
52502549	Topotecan inj 4mg		250	J9350	636	3	6/25/2015
52502556	Argatroban inj 250mg/2.5mL IV		250	C9121	636	3	5/24/2015
53101549	Morph analy tumor immuno qn	88360	310	88360	310	3	4/25/2015
53100004	Inshu lybrid each probe	88365	310	88365	310	3	7/3/2015
53101143	Em diagnostic	88348	312	88348	312	3	8/14/2014
53101150	Morphometric analy skel muscle	88355	312	88355	312	3	7/21/2015
53101168	Morphometric analy tumor	88358	312	88358	312	3	7/13/2015
53101176	Tissue in situ hybridization	88365	312	88365	312	3	8/8/2015
53600540	Inj wrist arthrogram-sur	25246	360	25246	360	3	7/15/2015
53600557	Inj wrist arthrogram-sur-bl	25246–50	360	25246–50	360	3	3/12/2015
54100144	MDI treatment, initial	94640	410	94640	410	3	7/8/2015
54100128	Continuous spag	94640	410	94640	410	3	6/15/2014
54100060	IPPB tx, subsequent	94640	410	94640	410	3	5/16/2014
54100037	IPPB therapy, initial	94640	410	94640	410	3	8/1/2014
54100011	Pentamadine aerosol tx	94640	410	94640	410	3	7/26/2014
57400186	Simp/comp pl gen w/o reprogram	95970	740	95970	740	3	7/13/2014
57400194	Simp pl gen w/reprogram	95971	740	95971	740	3	8/8/2014

Table 5.4. Sample CDM (Continued)

57400202	Cx brain pl gen w/rpg 1st hr	95978	740	95978	740	3	7/15/2014
58000068	Hemoperfusion	90997	801	90997	801	3	3/12/2014
58200015	Incenter dialysis-ped op <12kg	90999	821	90999	821	3	7/8/2014
58200023	Incenter dialysis-ped op >24kg	90999	821	90999	821	3	6/15/2014
58200031	Incenter dialysis-ped OP 12–24	90999	821	90999	821	3	5/16/2014
58500000	Home CCPD daily charge-ped	90947	851	90947	851	3	8/1/2014
59201780	Electronic analy of CI 1st hr	95974	920	95974	920	3	7/26/2014
59201772	Electronic analy CI addl 30 min	95975	920	95975	920	3	6/25/2014

Table 5.5. Basic content of a charge description master (CDM)

Field	Description	Example
Charge code	The facility's unique identifier for the specific charge. A hospital with outpatient services may have tens of thousands of charge codes. The codes may be assigned sequentially, as needed. However, the more logical assignment strategy is to link the sequence to the responsible department.	54100243 In this example, 541 is the department code for respiratory services.
Item description	The facility's description for the charge. The description should adequately differentiate between similar charges. In other words, multiple charges may have similar or identical descriptions; however, the HCPCS codes or revenue codes for the various charges vary. Therefore, the charge descriptions must be reviewed and amended to make the distinctions among charges clear.	Pulm Rehab 1 on 1 per 15 min. *versus* Pulm Rehab Therap Proc Grp
General ledger (GL) key	This code links the individual charge to the facility's accounting system.	3 = gross patient charges
Revenue code	The four-digit Medicare billing reference. These codes flow through to the UB (75.4–FL 42). Medicare guidelines suggest that the revenue code for a particular charge reflect the roll-up to the facility's cost report.	0410—General Classification Respiratory Service Detail: 041X is Respiratory Services 0—General classification (Respiratory SVC) 2—Inhalation Services (Inhalation SVC) 3—Hyperbaric Oxygen Therapy (Hyperbaric O_2) 9—Other Respiratory Services (Other Respir SVS)

Table 5.5. Basic content of a charge description master (CDM) (Continued)

Insurance code mapping (Mapping is also often referred to as *pointers* because the CDM is built to point to specific coding scenarios for a specific payer. This may also include different hard-coded modifier options by payer.)	These fields enable the assignment of multiple HCPCS codes and revenue codes to a single charge code. Medicare may require a specific HCPCS code for a charge, whereas a commercial payer may require a different code.	54100243 INS Code A payers require CPT code 97110, which is a nonspecific therapy code. INS Code B payers require HCPCS code G0238, which is specifically respiratory therapy.
Activity date	The effective date of the most current change. As a CDM matures, there are multiple changes that occur. Prices change, CPT codes change, and some charges become obsolete. The CDM should accommodate all of the above. For example, if a HCPCS code is replaced, the CDM should have the old data available for research and printing of old claims, but the new HCPCS code would fill the field in all claims after the date changed. So, the activity date reflects the most recent update, but there will be additional fields for the effective date or the expiration date of certain charges.	5/24/2008
Charge	This is the facility's gross charge for the service represented by the charge code. As described in chapter 2, the gross charge for a service is the same for all payers. Adjustments to charges, due to contractual arrangements and other discounts, are made on the back end.	$135

the system posts the multiple charges that are associated with the activity. Exploding charges will not work in all settings or for all payers, but it is an option for some organizations. The concept of exploding charges is also used when a hospital bills out both the facility (UB-04) and the physician (CMS-1500) charges. Medicare allows split billing by hospitals for facility and physician charges in which the UB captures the facility component with a revenue code (that is, clinic code revenue code 510) and a modifier signifying the claim is only for facility charges, while the CMS-1500 captures the physician charges.

Chargemaster Maintenance

The chargemaster requires continual maintenance to ensure that documentation and billing are accurate. The CDM must be updateable, and, because prices and other details change over time, the CDM must accommodate not only the current charge detail but also historical detail.

The finance department can use the CDM to increase charges and thus increase revenue. Charge increases are generally made on an annual basis, but they can be made as frequently as necessary to align the CDM with charges within their given market. Changes to charges in the CDM require a complex analysis, whether performed internally or outsourced to a consulting firm, of charge volumes for each service line, including reimbursement rates by payers that allow for a percentage of billed or billed eligible inpatient or outpatient charges as a reimbursement methodology; this analysis must also incorporates any managed care payer CDM increase thresholds contract provision clauses. These clauses often have a threshold or charge increase limit of 3 percent to 5 percent. Further, most state Medicaid and managed Medicaid programs require that a hospital notify the payer within a specific time frame that a CDM increase is taking place, for example, no less than 60 days prior to the intended effective date. Medicaid will then calculate a new cost-to-charge (CCR) ratio that the hospital will be paid for outpatient services. Medicaid generally does not allow any CDM increases. CDM policies should be verified with each state's Medicaid division. The CCR is based on the outpatient portion of the Medicaid cost report that was discussed in detail in chapter 2.

As of January 1, 2016, claims must distinguish place-of-service (POS) 22, which designates that services were rendered in an on-campus hospital outpatient setting, from POS code 19, which designates that services were rendered in an off-campus hospital outpatient setting; furthermore, these POS codes must have any necessary modifiers to signify that the claim is for the physician component only. Prior to January 4, 2016, only POS code 22 was used for both scenarios. This change was implemented to facilitate Medicaid and other payers' need for greater specificity in the hospital setting. While Medicare does not distinguish between the on-campus and off-campus settings for payment purposes, other payers, such as Medicaid, do (CMS 2015b). However, Medicare does make the on-campus versus off-campus distinction, which is based on the hospital's Medicare participation documentation of which site is the main site and which sites are ancillary or satellite, for administrative purposes. This recent POS change highlights why revenue cycle practitioners need to pay close attention to CMS transmittals, as updates to the patient access modules or systems and the billing modules or systems, as well as staff education, are required to address such changes.

Maintenance of the CDM is a multidisciplinary activity. For example, the HIM department knows the clinical codes; the patient accounts department knows what the general billing edit issues are for the facility; the pharmacy department knows the drugs and their costs; the finance department knows the associated charge formulas and general ledger codes; and managed care knows the payer billing policies. Pharmacy staff cannot realistically update the radiology department's data, nor can finance staff update charges without knowledge of underlying costs. To coordinate the update effort, a single department, usually the budgeting and reimbursement or managed care department within the finance division, should be assigned responsibility for ensuring timely updates. The finance department then should enlist the assistance of other disciplines, including HIM. Update frequency depends on the data element to be updated, but the CDM certainly should be updated whenever underlying costs or codes change. For example, pharmacy charges may be updated every time inventory is replenished. The entire CDM must be reviewed at least annually (Davis 2010, 792–793).

Many hospitals use CDM committees or teams, consisting of members from departments hospital-wide, to establish and maintain an accurate chargemaster description. Ambulatory payment classification (APC) and DRG reimbursement methodologies and healthcare technology are changing rapidly, requiring the CDM be revised on a continual basis. A team approach will maximize reimbursement and make maintenance process more efficient and effective than an individual approach by implementing changes quickly and ensuring that all departments affected by the change receive adequate advance notice. At an absolute minimum, a CDM must be updated annually to reflect the CPT/HCPCS code updates, which have typically taken place each January 1st. Most healthcare facilities add, delete, or change services frequently and prefer to update the CDM continually; thus, the CDM maintenance team meets regularly, often monthly.

A CDM team will require that a facility expend resources, therefore incurring costs. A charge-master team should be appointed by carefully selecting interdepartmental clinical and hospital managers. Employees, end users, and technical staff may also be included on a permanent or an ad-hoc basis. Team members should be carefully selected for their specific knowledge and expertise as well as their vested interest in the specific charges. Representatives from laboratory, radiology, HIM, and patient financial services, as well as staff from clinical areas such as surgery, are important to include. Member education and cross training are important first steps for each and every member. For example, clinical directors and finance personnel are typically unfamiliar with coding policies and procedures, and HIM professionals will need to acquire a more thorough understanding of billing activities and systems (Drach et al. 2001).

Every team member needs to know which CPT/HCPCS codes are hard coded and which are soft coded. When codes are *hard coded*, the HCPCS code is automatically assigned by the information system based on a charge code. *Soft coding* refers to HCPCS code assignment and subsequent data entry into the billing system by HIM coders after record review. For the soft-coded records, the team should have a master list of who codes the various types of claims. Clarification in this area will reduce double billing, missed coding, and subsequent payer denials and lowers the facility's risk for fraud and abuse charges.

Another important component in maintaining the facility's CDM is reviewing claim denials. Organizations need to develop a comprehensive system for investigating and correcting claim denials. Often, a facility corrects these problems on an individual case-by-case basis. Through appropriate auditing, analysis, and communication, the source of problem(s) can be identified and corrective action taken. In many cases, the source of the problem can be traced back to the CDM, and the amount of time expended by billing and HIM personnel correcting these problems is eliminated by making the appropriate CDM updates or changes. Communication and information sharing among team members are also important to improve efficiency and reduce work redundancy.

One of the disadvantages of a poorly selected team or committee is that it can take longer to make decisions and implement changes. This is the antithesis of one of the major goals for using the team approach. Therefore, the leader, or chair, of the team should have strong leadership and project management skills. The leader must coordinate all team activities, such as scheduling meetings, assigning individual member tasks, ensuring that the project is completed as scheduled, and following-up on any implementations or recommendations.

The leader must also establish formal lines of communication to distribute information regarding proposed changes both within the committee and among important departments that may not have team representation. The leader must also establish communication lines to disseminate important information contained in Medicare bulletins and transmittals and the National Correct Coding Initiative (NCCI). A specific procedure, including request forms, should be established to allow department directors to submit chargemaster change requests for new, deleted, or revised procedures and services.

Bundling Issues

Charges for echocardiograms are a good example of the type of routine CDM changes that a facility might need. Prior to January 2009, echocardiograms with Doppler wave spectral display and color flow velocity were charged using three separate codes:

* 93307—Echocardiography, transthoracic
* 93318—Doppler echocardiography, pulsed wave and/or continuous wave with spectral display
* 93325—Doppler echocardiography color flow velocity

Each procedure had a separate charge code, and the facility might have opted to set up a single charge that exploded into the three charges if there were numerous cases in which all three procedures were done. As of January 1, 2009, a comprehensive code (93306) was added to CPT to bundle all three procedures. The facility would then have had to make the old exploding charge obsolete as of January 1, 2009, and create a new charge code for the bundled service. The individual codes are still valid, so those would remain. For services after the effective date, use of the exploding charge to produce the three codes would be incorrect and the claim would fail.

Another example of unbundling is the potential conflict between the codes associated with CDM charges (hard-coded charges) and the codes assigned in the HIM department (soft-coded charges). Generally, an HIM coder assigns a specific CPT code for a surgical procedure whereas the surgery department may have entered codes to reflect charges for the surgical suite and individual items used. In some cases, however, a procedure may be added to the charge in the clinical area. For example, radiology codes, including interventional radiology, may be assigned in the radiology department *or* attached to the CDM. The HIM coder must be alert to this potential duplication, which would result in double billing for the same procedure. Another type of error can occur if both a CDM code and an HIM code are validly assigned. Because some multiple codes cannot be billed together or require a combination code or modifier, this bill will fail if the unbundling is not corrected. Situations like this should appear on a prebilling error report so that the error can be evaluated and corrected before billing occurs. The HIM department is a logical area to undertake this evaluation because the error can be corrected and the coder remediated as needed. Claims processing and error reports are discussed in more detail in chapter 7.

Timeliness

Charges must be recorded for the date of service, which in turn must take place during the dates of service stated on the uniform bill (UB-04). Charges that are recorded for dates outside the UB-04 range will cause the bill to fail. Charges that are recorded after the date of service are late charges. Since one of the main purposes of a bill hold is to capture late charges, it is acceptable (although not best practice) to record charges up to the end of the bill-hold period. Charges recorded after the bill-hold period are problematic, as discussed in chapter 6.

Another issue with respect to timeliness is the handling of claims around the time of coding changes. In the previous echocardiography bundling example, an account with a discharge date of December 31, 2008, would be correctly billed with the exploding charge, and a claim with a discharge date of January 1, 2009, would be correctly billed with the bundled code. However, due to bill-hold requirements, both charges could theoretically drop and bill on the same day in January.

Internal controls to ensure timely recording of charges are critical for efficient revenue cycle management. Clinical departments that have difficulty ensuring that charges are posted on a timely basis should examine their workflow. Lean methodologies for performance improvement are optimal in this scenario. The goal is to develop processes that yield the highest degree of timeliness and accuracy in charge capture with the fewest steps and least amount effort. For instance, consider a manual charge-capture system that requires multiple individuals to list individual charges by hand on a pick list or other paper charge-capture form. Bar coding supplies and scanning them for use at point of care can reduce error and minimize effort in the clinical area. However, the set-up for such a system is time consuming and the cost can be prohibitive. The cost justification must take into consideration the time savings in charge capture as well as the reduction in time required to make corrections and rebill.

Accuracy

The existence of a charge code does not inherently mean that using that code is correct in every situation. Clinical department personnel who are responsible for charging must be educated as to the appropriate charges for services. Going back to the previous echocardiography bundling example, personnel who were unaware of the CPT code charge would continue to drop the out-of-date charges until they were informed otherwise. Furthermore, the quantities of individual charges must be correct, which places additional responsibilities on the clinical department management to ensure that charges are not only complete but accurate. Compliance with correct coding guidelines and correct billing guidelines is inherently part of the charging responsibility.

Check Your Understanding 5.2.

1. What is a chargemaster and why is it important?

2. How often does a chargemaster get updated?

3. What is an exploding charge and how is it affected by bundling?

Internal Controls

In any industry, internal controls must be in place to safeguard assets and to ensure compliance with policies and procedures. Internal controls may be designed to prevent the theft of cash or to ensure that a patient receives the correct medication. The three major categories of internal controls are preventive, detective, and corrective controls (Davis 2010, 796).

Preventive Controls

Preventive controls are implemented at the front end of a process. They are specifically designed to stop an incorrect or inappropriate activity. For example, computer data-entry validation of a date would prevent someone from entering "13" for a month or "45" for a day. Preventive controls in patient access help registrars identify missing and potentially erroneous data.

In many cases, preventive controls are time consuming and not cost-effective. If every registrar had to stop and correct every single error or omission at the point of registration, the number of patients who could be registered in a day would be quite small. Preventive controls are typically developed and implemented for critical process points in which the error would cause a failure of the function or other major problem. For example, three-point patient identification is a preventive control that helps stop the administration of medications to the wrong patient. If preventive controls are not cost-effective or practical, then detective and corrective controls must be developed and implemented to find and fix errors.

Detective Controls

Detective controls are put in place to find errors that may have been made during a process. Routine coding-quality audits and registration audits are examples of detective controls. Detective controls can be more cost effective than preventive controls in finding errors, partly because the detective process is specifically designed to find specific errors or anomalies in data. Detective controls are appropriate when errors can be found before they result in a failure of the function or other major problem. Therefore, the most efficient detective controls in the revenue cycle process take place prior to billing. Once the bill has dropped, the cost of reviewing and correcting errors increases. Because detective controls only find errors, they must be accompanied by corrective controls to fix the errors.

Corrective Controls

Corrective controls are designed to fix problems that have already occurred. They are most often associated with a preceding detective control that identified the problem. In the revenue cycle process, corrective controls apply to any modification of the demographic, financial, or clinical data that result in a more accurate claim. Corrective controls apply to registration activities, such as completing a registration as well as obtaining payer authorization for the encounter if the authorization was not done before registration. The process for completing health records post-discharge is also a corrective control.

From a billing perspective, there are few errors that cannot be corrected before the claim is sent to the payer. One error that cannot be corrected is the completion of a service that will not be reimbursed. Errors that cannot always be corrected include theft of assets and theft of data. Otherwise, errors that are detected can be corrected, and doing so within the bill-hold period is generally less costly than trying to make corrections retrospectively. An important application of detective and corrective controls is the review and reconciliation of orders.

Reconciling Orders

Clinical departments that are responsible for executing orders, such as radiology, laboratory, and pharmacy, must reconcile the number and type of orders with the actual services provided. This reconciliation should be done daily. Daily reconciliation facilitates early detection of open orders, duplicate orders, and missing orders. All clinical services must be preceded by a physician order, which may be documented electronically or by paper script. Failure to detect and correct errors at this stage will result in missing charges, delayed billing, rebilling, or denials for medical necessity.

Open Orders

Open orders are orders that have been placed but have not been completed. For example, the physician writes an order for an x-ray of the foot. The nurse takes the order from the physician order sheet, conveys that order to radiology, and marks it complete on the order sheet. However, radiology has three additional steps: perform the order, record the charge for the test, and provide results of the examination.

There are several controls in place on the clinical side to ensure that ordered tests are performed. Not the least of these controls is the physician who, having ordered an x-ray, is looking for the results.

Canceled Orders

Sometimes, orders are cancelled, perhaps because the patient is discharged prior to the execution of the order, the medical necessity of the test is re-evaluated, or the patient refuses the test or drug. Both the ordering department and the receiving department must ensure that the orders are canceled in the organization's computer system. Failure to cancel an order in a timely manner will result in wasted time, effort, and sometimes supplies as the receiving department attempts to fulfill the order.

Results

The results of the order (laboratory test results, radiological findings, or therapy notes) are the clinical documentation that supports the charge. Just because the test was ordered does not mean that it was completed. The physician order is a clue to look for the test results, not proof that the test occurred. The results documentation is critical for defense of reimbursement denials. Therefore, release-of-information personnel in the HIM department should ensure that they are knowledgeable regarding the storage and retention of all test results.

If test results are in the EHR, how are they printed or downloaded for release to a payer? If they are retained in the testing department, how accessible are they? If the test was ordered and it seems to have been performed, but the results are not in the expected place, is there a backup method for determining whether the test was really performed and obtaining the results? For example, there may be an ancillary support system in the department that maintains all test results. These are questions that need to be answered so that the appropriate documentation can be obtained quickly. Figure 5.1 shows a documentation-and-retention questionnaire that can be used to obtain the answers to these questions. (An electronic example of this questionnaire is included in the book's online resources.)

Figure 5.1.   Sample documentation-and-retention questionnaire and data capture tool

Documentation-and-Retention Questionnaire

Please complete this questionnaire and return it by _____ to _____ in the Health Information Management Department.

Department/Section: _____

Location: _____

Contact: _____ Telephone #: _____

1. Do you generate patient-specific reports in your area?   ☐ Yes   ☐ No
    If No, please stop here and return questionnaire to Health Information Management.

2. For each of the following types of reports, please check all that apply to your area, identify the documents, and indicate how they are retained.

	Name of Report	Filed in Department	Generated and Stored Electronically. Please Specify System	Scanned and Stored Electronically. Please Specify System	Delivered to Health Information Management
Individual Reports					
Images					
Complete patient record					

3. How far back can you access electronically stored reports? Please specify system(s)
    _____

4. How many months or years of individual reports do you have on site? _____

5. Where do you archive individual reports on site? _____

6. How many months or years of images do you have on site? _____

7. Where do you archive images on site? _____

Figure 5.1. Sample documentation-and-retention questionnaire and data capture tool (Continued)

8. How many months or years of complete patient records do you have on site? _____

9. Where do you archive complete patient records on site? _____

10. Does Health Information Management handle *all* of your on-demand requests for release of information? (Including patients, legal, insurance, and other external requests)
    ☐ Yes ☐ No

11. If the answer to question 10 is No, please describe your release-of-information process in the space below.

    _____

    _____

Back-End Reporting

Key performance indicators (KPIs) are essential to the financial success of a hospital. Several of the KPIs discussed in this chapter need to be a part of any revenue cycle team's KPI dashboards (see example in chapter 1), which are reports of process measures that assist with strategic planning. Data from these reports can be compiled into a spreadsheet or on a page in the organization's intranet for quick reference. A dashboard may include the discharged, no final bill (DNFB) report, a late-charges report, carve-out reports by revenue code (based on contract rate schedules and CDM build), and payer rules that affect reimbursement. Each of these reports allows the revenue cycle team to see what, if any, issues are preventing the submission of clean claims to payers within the bill-hold period.

Routine Statistical Reports

The DNFB report is one of the most important KPIs monitored by revenue cycle teams. This report is reviewed to identify the number of accounts that are past the bill-hold period because of late charges, the number of accounts that need to be combined based on specific Medicare or payer rules, and the number of accounts that cannot be billed out because HIM needs additional documentation from a department or the physician to finish coding the record. Thorough, complete documentation is key to HIM's ability to code an account for billing. Missing documentation accounts for a large percentage of accounts being on the DNFB past the close of the bill-hold period.

A late-charge report should be generated daily and shared with the individual clinical areas to resolve any late-charge issues. If late charges are included on the KPI dashboard, the dollar amount would be captured at a high level (the total charges by number of days out from date of service), but if a more significant issue exists, there may be a need to report by department and number of days out with total charges. The designated person in each clinical department should explain and justify the late charges. If the late charges are not resolved within the bill-hold period, then a corrected claim needs to be submitted by patient financial services. This correction will cause the account to re-adjudicate within the hospital's reimbursement or contract management system to ensure that the expected reimbursement is accurately reflected in the system. Late charges need to be handled in this manner so they make it into the account; the account can then be updated to correctly reflect open accounts receivable. (See chapter 2 for a discussion of accounting terms.) Running daily reports will allow the revenue cycle team to determine which clinical areas need updated training on charge entry or may simply need a backup plan for when the designated charge-entry person is out of the office. As previously mentioned; if late charges are entered after the bill-hold period, the delay will cause claims management issues (to be addressed in chapter 6) for patient financial services.

Carve-out reports are another area of significant importance to the revenue cycle team. These reports help to ensure that all high-cost drugs and implantables are captured on the claim. This documentation is particularly important not just for cost analysis but also because these items may be separately payable, depending on the payer. These reports should be run by *International Classification of Diseases, Tenth Revision, Procedure Coding System (ICD-10-PCS)* code. If a chart is coded to document that a pacemaker was implanted, then there should be a corresponding charge with revenue code 275 for the high-cost implantable (the pacemaker). In the past, charts had to be manually audited to capture missing high-cost items that are carved out in the payer contracts. Looking at accounts based on coding done by HIM allows for a lesser degree of manual intervention. Carve-out reports should be run for all payers, but special attention should be given to those payers that additionally pay the hospital for high-cost drugs or implantables (such payments are known as carved-out payments). Often, there is a threshold associated with the carved-out items in the contract. Contract wording varies, but the following represents typical language: "High implantables billed out under revenue codes 271–279 that cost the hospital more than $10,000 per item will be paid XX% of invoice cost in addition to the negotiated per diem." Because these items cost the hospital substantial sums, the facility will want to be reimbursed, at a minimum, for the items' cost in addition to the per diem. The second part of this KPI is whether or not the facility was paid correctly. This topic will be discussed further in chapter 7.

Compliance-Related Reports

The revenue cycle team should review which rules from Medicare, Medicaid, and other payers affect the hospital's reimbursement. Reports are needed to track those CMS rules that other national- and state-based payers currently have in place or are trying to adopt through contractual or policy and procedure changes, including the following: the three-day payment window (CMS 2014a), readmission within 30 days (CMS 2014b), and hospital-acquired conditions (HACs) (CMS 2014c).

The three-day payment window requires that a hospital include in the inpatient bill any outpatient services related to the inpatient admission that have occurred at the facility within three days of the admission or discharge. If a hospital uses one name and one tax identification number for its freestanding surgery center or physical therapy center and its main acute-care facility, then all inpatient care and outpatient services directly related to the inpatient diagnosis need to be included on the admission bill. The three-day payment window is not a rule many providers agree to allow payers to implement for commercial product lines (nongovernmental contracts).

Readmissions must also be included in compliance-related reports. CMS is in the process of adopting a readmission within 30 days of inpatient stay (discharge) rule through the Readmission Reduction Program. With the goal of reducing readmissions, hospitals have begun to dedicate employees in their case management or care management departments to identifying and tracking patients who have been readmitted for the same condition within 30 days of discharge. Readmission reports can be used to identify patients, who may not have been identified prior to discharge, in need of postdischarge tracking by discharge-follow-up nurses or social workers. Tracking is intended to ensure that patients are compliant with their doctor's home care instructions and may involve ensuring that patients take their medications or attend scheduled follow-up physician appointments. As part of this Readmission Reduction Program, Medicare provides a list of diagnoses that fall within the 30-day readmissions rule, including acute exacerbation of chronic obstructive pulmonary disease (COPD), total hip arthroplasty, and total knee arthroplasty. Reports that include the designated diagnoses should be generated daily to ensure that accounts have been combined as needed prior to billing; they also allow the hospital to track the costs that payers are not reimbursing.

Medicare does not allow hospitals to increase the DRG payment for a hospital stay associated with certain HACs, such as a traumatic fracture that was not present on admission. Medicare has initiated a HAC-reduction program as part of the Affordable Care Act (CMS 2014d). Some managed care payers are taking this rule one step further and denying all payment on an account with a specified HAC. The HAC report is based on the specific codes that signify the patient has a HAC. CMS has published a list of these conditions, and most commercial payers are also incorporating that list into their contracts to negatively impact reimbursement. The HAC reports should be shared with the chief nursing officer (CNO) and chief operation officer (COO) as well as risk-management leadership to confirm that the hospital is making any necessary changes to ensure patient safety and reduce the incidence of HACs. The revenue cycle team needs to be aware of expected reimbursement losses due to HACs. The HAC reports provide an opportunity to incorporate clinical leadership into the revenue cycle team discussions. The CNO or COO can explain to the revenue cycle team what corrective action is being taken to reduce HACs and, therefore, increase reimbursement to the hospital.

Special Considerations for Specific Practice Settings

All settings have much the same transaction flow—register the patient, examine him or her, document relevant data, order services, and treat—but documentation and charge capture issues vary based on the billing requirements and the volume of transactions in the particular setting. Whereas inpatient documentation and orders are typically completed as a single case, outpatient documentation can be less finite. For example, inpatient test results are typically reviewed and acted on during the episode of care, but physician office visits may be complete in the absence of such documentation. Further, physician offices likely do not have volumes of open orders to review at the end of the day.

Inpatient Settings

Whether the patient is an inpatient or an outpatient is a key issue in the inpatient setting. Although the definitions are clear, the actual documentation does not always reflect the level of clarity or direction that is necessary to make a definitive decision. Historically, acute-care hospitals have wrestled with unclear documentation such as an order to "admit for observation," which created ambiguity as to whether the patient was an inpatient (admitted) or an outpatient (in observation status). The evolving two-midnight rule should assist with resolving this issue. Further, the medical necessity that drives the level of care is not always well documented. Clinical documentation programs are proving valuable in this regard. The timing of charge capture can be problematic, in light of the volume of charges that are posted and the decentralization of the review and validation of daily charges—hence the need for internal controls, order reconciliation, and back-end monitoring of activities.

Outpatient Settings

For outpatient services, maintenance of the CDM is a key issue. When setting up the charge, the proper revenue code must be assigned as well as the correct CPT/HCPCS code. Changes to CPT/HCPCS must be identified, and the CDM must be updated accurately.

Proving medical necessity can be problematic because physician scripts do not always contain the appropriate ICD-10-CM code. Patient access registrars cannot be expected to realize that a CT scan is not justified by unspecified anemia. Without front-end medical-necessity edits, especially for Medicare patients, these errors will not be caught until the bill drops unless the outpatient services department takes a proactive role in identifying and correcting these errors. Since the department needs a medical reason for the test in the first place, it seems reasonable that they should also look at the admitting codes to see whether they make sense. Timely resolution of this issue will help the bill drop faster.

Physician Practices

Physicians typically maintain one record per patient—accounts not necessarily reflected in the record. If the records are stored in a problem-oriented format, it may be difficult to pull together the documentation to support a particular claim. An EHR solves these problems. Charge capture in a physician office, absent an EHR, may be supported by an encounter form (also known as a superbill)—a document on which the physician can check off the patient's diagnosis and the procedures performed, including office visit time.

Physician billing for inpatient services may require copies of part of the inpatient record. The HIM department must have policies and procedures in place to handle the documentation requests from physicians for copies of progress notes. In an EHR, the physicians can potentially download the documentation themselves. However, if this documentation is still in paper format, the photocopying may be a burden to HIM. The hospital must identify the scope of this issue and determine what arrangements best suit all parties concerned.

Check Your Understanding 5.3.

1. What are the three main types of internal controls?

2. What is the purpose of reconciling orders?

3. What are the key issues related to back-end reporting?

References

Centers for Medicare and Medicaid Services (CMS). 2015a. Fact Sheet: Two Midnight Rule. https://www.cms.gov/Newsroom/MediaReleaseDatabase/Fact-sheets/2015-Fact-sheets-items/2015-07-01-2.html.

Centers for Medicare and Medicaid Services (CMS). 2015b. CMS Manual System, Pub 100-04 Medicare Claims Processing, Transmittal 3315. https://www.cms.gov/Regulations-and-Guidance/Guidance/Transmittals/Downloads/R3315CP.pdf.

Centers for Medicare and Medicaid Services (CMS). 2014a. 3 Day Payment Window. https://www.cms.gov/Medicare/Medicare-Fee-for-Service-Payment/AcuteInpatientPPS/Three_Day_Payment_Window.html.

Centers for Medicare and Medicaid Services (CMS). 2014b. Readmission Reductions Program. https://www.cms.gov/medicare/medicare-fee-for-service-payment/acuteinpatientpps/readmissions-reduction-program.html.

Centers for Medicare and Medicaid Services (CMS). 2014c. Hospital Acquired Conditions (Present on Admission Indicator). https://www.cms.gov/Medicare/Medicare-Fee-for-Service-Payment/HospitalAcqCond/index.html.

Centers for Medicare and Medicaid Services (CMS). 2014d. Hospital Acquired Conditions Reduction Program. https://www.cms.gov/Medicare/Medicare-Fee-for-Service-Payment/AcuteInpatientPPS/HAC-Reduction-Program.html.

Davis, N. 2010. Financial management. Chapter 25 in *Health Information Management: Concepts, Principles, and Practice*, 3rd ed. Edited by K.M. LaTour and S. Eichenwald Maki. Chicago: AHIMA.

Drach, M., A. Davis, and C. Sagrati. 2001. Ten steps to successful chargemaster reviews. *Journal of AHIMA* 72(1): 421–448.

Hess, P. 2015. Assessing clinical documentation. Chapter 5 in *Clinical Documentation Improvement: Principles and Practice.* Chicago: AHIMA.

Record Completion and Coding

Learning Objectives

- Examine the impact of the record completion process on revenue cycle.
- Illustrate the health information management (HIM) department's role in creating a clean claim.
- Understand how to develop an effective coding quality process.

Key Terms

- Backlog
- Hospital-acquired condition (HAC)
- Late charges
- Physician query process policy
- Postdischarge processing
- Present on admission (POA)
- Probationary period
- Revenue code

The health information management (HIM) department has played an important role in the revenue cycle for the past three decades through coding and other core functions. The activities in the HIM department all support the revenue cycle, either by supporting coding or by ensuring the timely release of information needed for billing. Efficient postdischarge processing is therefore a key revenue cycle component.

Postdischarge Processing

Postdischarge processing is a traditional role of the HIM department. Whether the record is entirely electronic, entirely paper, or a hybrid combination of the two, the HIM department is charged with ensuring that the record is complete, coded, abstracted, properly stored, and accessible. The procedures by which these activities occur vary significantly depending on the level of point-of-care electronic data capture.

Timely Record Availability

Very little postdischarge processing can occur if the HIM department has not obtained control of the complete health record. Policies and procedures must be in place both in the HIM department as well as facility-wide to ensure that records are obtained in a timely fashion.

As long as any significant portion of the patient record is paper-based at point of care, HIM will need to obtain physical control of the hard-copy documentation. HIM must not only get the record and check it in but also ensure that all possible components have been received. For example, if a primarily electronic health record (EHR) has components that may or may not be present in paper format, such as certain patient consent documents, physician documentation, and diagnostic testing reports, the EHR must be analyzed to determine what, if anything, is missing. Of course, in a completely electronic health record, access is not the issue; instead, the activity becomes the issue. Records may be in process for analysis and being completed by the clinician simultaneously. Systems that support the linking of the analysis to the deficiency (missing or incomplete documentation) will most efficiently reflect the current state of the record's completeness.

Traditionally, patient records were not in the control of the HIM department until clinical personnel who directly cared for the patient completed their documentation. However, with the expansion of the Centers for Medicare and Medicaid Services (CMS) prospective payment system (PPS) and the increase in the percentage of managed care plans across all payers, the competing interests increasingly involve completion of required minimum data set (MDS 3.0) filings as well as utilization and reviews, such as surgical case review. Therefore, immediate HIM access to the patient's record for coding becomes a challenge in a paper-based environment. Because uncoded records appear on the discharged, no final bill (DNFB) report with a notation to that effect, facilities must make some effort to ensure that all parties are aware of the reason for coding delays. Because many claims cannot be processed without certifying days or completing data set forms, clearly identifying why accounts remain on the DNFB may be sufficient.

In more aggressive claims-processing scenarios, incomplete paperwork may not be an adequate explanation for noncoding of records. Particularly in a five-day bill hold, few reasons plausibly excuse the failure to complete paperwork on a timely basis. Therefore, it is imperative that the HIM department develop and maintain excellent relationships with all relevant clinical departments and encourage them to establish policies and procedures that support postdischarge processing within the appropriate bill-hold time frame. Birth certificate preparation for infants born in the hospital is one example. If the clinical department processes birth certificates prior to releasing the infant's chart, any delay in this process holds up coding. Filing of a birth certificate is necessary; however, it need not precede final billing. Therefore, it is reasonable to ask the clinical area to send all newborn records to HIM prior to the expiration of the bill hold for check-in and coding. The records can then be checked out and returned to the clinical area for birth certificate processing.

This same arrangement can be made for any department that needs to have access to the records immediately postdischarge. If both coding and other processing affect final billing, the record can be placed on hold for final billing. In this manner, the record is then appropriately flagged. Sometimes, HIM personnel can hold the bill either through a computer system function or simply by not coding it; otherwise, the patient accounting department will have to be notified to hold the bill to prevent a final bill from dropping. The advantage of having a specific computer system function to segregate or flag these accounts is that they can be automatically identified on a routine error report, rather than HIM personnel having to manually prepare an exception list for DNFB reporting purposes.

Backlogs

For the purpose of this discussion, a backlog is an existing volume of processing that has already exceeded the ability of the HIM department to process it on a timely basis in the normal course of business. The backlog that most obviously affects the revenue cycle is coding. However, depending on the process flow in the department, any process that precedes coding has a similar impact.

In an electronic health record, the primary backlog involves the completion of dictations. Surgical cases should not be coded without a pathology report if tissue was sent for analysis and the availability of an operative report is optimal.

Incomplete Records—Interacting with Physicians

According to Joint Commission standards and CMS Conditions of Participation, a physician must complete an inpatient record within 30 days of discharge (Joint Commission 2015a; CMS 2015a). Some state regulations as well as individual facility medical staff bylaws, rules, and regulations may shorten that time period. However, even a 14-day completion window for physician records is too long to satisfy the typical bill-hold period of 3 to 5 days postdischarge. If a chart cannot be coded because information from a physician is needed, coding staff must be assertive in making their needs known. The pressure to drop bills in a timely manner is acute, and HIM struggle with the conflicting priorities of speedy processing versus accuracy and completeness. Ultimately, however, dropping a correct bill late is a better practice than dropping bills hastily and rebilling the corrections. Thus, fostering excellent relationships with physicians to facilitate timely chart completion is essential. In a completely electronic health record system, it is entirely reasonable to expect chart completion within the bill-hold period.

Physician Completion

The face sheet, discharge summary, operative report, and pathology report are the most common deficiencies that delay coding.

A patient's electronic record may effectively summarize the diagnoses for the coder via computer-assisted coding (CAC) software. When an inpatient is discharged, a discharge summary that details the patient's reason for hospitalization, treatment, outcome of hospitalization, discharge disposition, and discharge instructions is required (Joint Commission 2015b; CMS 2015a). In a paper or hybrid record, physicians may also be expected to summarize their assessments on a face sheet. In many cases, such a summary is merely a formality, particularly if the documentation in the rest of the record is thorough and complete and the discharge summary is completed.

Although coders are trained to take into consideration the totality of physician documentation, the discharge summary helps them understand the episode of care from the physician's perspective. The quality of discharge summaries may be an issue if they are routinely dictated by clinicians other than the attending physician. Periodic audits of the completeness and accuracy of discharge summaries are a universally good compliance practice. However, in the presence of an alternative dictator program, they become essential.

The operative report is important when coding complex procedures. Although the postoperative progress note and perioperative record generally contain sufficient detail to enable the coder to identify the procedure performed, the level of detail needed to code with specificity is only found in the operative report. The operative report must be completed as soon as possible after the completion of the procedure (Joint Commission 2015c). Most deficiencies of this type are not identified and flagged until quantitative analysis, which may take place after coding. If tardy operative reports are problematic, earlier identification may be required. The HIM department may want to partner with other relevant departments to develop and implement a performance improvement plan to increase compliance. Tracking the completion of operative reports from the point of care (in this case, the procedure) better highlights the issue than waiting until after discharge.

If a specimen obtained during an operative procedure was sent to the pathology department for review, it is generally essential for the coder to wait for a pathology report before coding the record. In this situation, the record can be coded for all other conditions; however, assignment of the final diagnosis related to the operative episode must be deferred. Because some specimens must be sent out for analysis, the wait for the pathology report can be long. It is possible that the report may not be available for a matter of months. Consultation with the pathology department and the surgeon may yield a high level of confidence in the expected pathology results, particularly if previous biopsies are available and documented in the current record. In other cases, final coding will not be possible until the results are received. This is not to say that coders should just sit and wait. It is appropriate to follow-up with pathology to ensure timely receipt of the results.

Physician Query Procedures

Communication with physicians regarding completion or clarification of documentation essential to coding should be part of a standard **physician query process policy**. The online resources that accompany this book include AHIMA's *Practice Brief: Guidelines for Achieving a Compliant Query Practice* (AHIMA 2013).

The key to a successful query is to ensure that the physician responds by amending the clinical record as requested—for example, by providing documentation or clarification of the record. Queries may be electronic, which facilitates this process. If the query form is a part of the official record, then the physician may respond on the query form, but the response must be given completely in writing, including date and signature. This process is not optimum because the query form is not where the EHR should have been noted in the first place. For this reason, use of the query form should be discouraged except for clarifications. If the physician is asked to document a diagnosis or procedure that is not clearly present in the existing record, an amendment to the clinical record is suggested. In the past, the presence of laboratory values for low hemoglobin combined with the transfusion of packed cells was sufficient to code a diagnosis of anemia even in the absence of a stated diagnosis. However, this practice is no longer acceptable because CMS and payers expect the physician to review the labs and clearly document what the findings mean for the patient. If the physician seems to have identified and treated a condition without specifically identifying it in the clinical record, a postdischarge progress note to incorporate the diagnosis, a reference on the face sheet (if applicable), and a mention of the diagnosis in the discharge summary would be ideal. All entries must be properly authenticated. The extent to which this documentation is acceptable depends on the payer.

Delays and Refusals

For the most part, physicians want their documentation in the patient's record to be accurate. However, there are often delays in their responses to HIM-related queries, and some physicians are not willing to amend what they have already documented.

One way to communicate a query to a physician is to include the query as part of the quantitative analysis process. If analysis takes place promptly following coding—within a day or two—then the query form can be placed on the chart for the physician to complete. Assuming the physician routinely visits the HIM department for chart completion, the completed query and the chart can be returned to the coder in the normal course of chart processing. This somewhat idealized process can work very well if the physician is also notified immediately that there is a query waiting for review.

If the analysis function is delayed, then the coder will have a better result by contacting the physician directly with the query. A fax to the physician's office will work for this purpose. If it is possible to build a query function into the computer system, that would also work well. Oral communication is not acceptable for most queries, because amendment or completion of the record itself is usually necessary.

Occasionally, a physician will refuse to amend the record. For example, a physician operates on a patient to remove multiple skin tags and moles. On the face sheet, the physician records "mole." On review of the pathology report, the coder sees that the mole was really "malignant melanoma" and queries the physician, who then refuses to amend the documentation in the record. In these cases, it would be useful to have a physician-oriented documentation-improvement process with a procedure in place to refer such cases to a physician panel for review and counseling of the recalcitrant physician. Refusal to amend documentation is not just a revenue cycle issue. Certain diagnoses, such as congestive heart failure and acute myocardial infarction, are reportable for the Joint Commission's performance improvement core measures (Joint Commission 2014), and others, such as cancer, are reportable to certain registries. Failure to accurately record these diagnoses affects those activities.

Other Chart-Processing Delays

In a paper or heavily paper hybrid-record environment, processing delays can be caused by events that remove all or part of the chart from the normal postdischarge process. If the chart removal occurs prior to coding, the bill may be delayed. Common events that may delay processing include audit, utilization review (UR), clinical chart completion, and continuing patient care. The HIM department should have a policy and procedure in place for handling each of these issues. A fully implemented EHR alleviates these sorts of processing delays for the most part. Audits and continuing patient care will not stop a chart from being processed in an EHR. However, UR—the process of determining whether the medical care provided to a specific patient is necessary according to preestablished objective screening criteria—will still be a potential cause of processing delays, particularly with regard to the certification of days. Although postdischarge processing may continue, certain bills will not drop without certification. Use of an EHR should facilitate and, one hopes, streamline clinical chart completion.

Audits of recently discharged patients are usually internal. Since the payer has not yet been billed, a billing audit will not occur in this situation. However, the case may come up in a compliance or performance-improvement audit. Whenever possible, it is best to ask the auditor to visit the HIM department to perform the audit. The record can be tagged for easy retrieval and pulled when the auditor arrives. A colored flag on the folder notifies staff at what point in the process the record was pulled. Another method of tagging is to enclose the record in a brightly colored folder. If the auditor is not able or willing to visit the HIM department, the chart should be coded before it is sent for audit.

Utilization review is an important component of the revenue cycle. If the inpatient days of service are not authorized, the payer may refuse to reimburse the facility. Case-management or UR personnel review the length of stays continuously from admission to discharge; however, some residual tasks may take place postdischarge. Since some payers, such as Medicaid, may not be billed until the inpatient days have been certified, it is in everyone's best interest to ensure that UR has appropriate access to the records. Since UR is an ongoing issue, the best approach is to develop an excellent working relationship between the HIM department and UR or case-management staff so that a timely process may be established. For example, UR may notify HIM that the record is being held for review by leaving a card in the chart pick-up tray. This way, HIM can immediately "check out" the record to UR for tracking purposes and follow-up within 24 hours to obtain the record. Timely follow-up is essential to ensure that all processes are completed prior to the bill release. Alternatively, UR staff may be willing to visit the HIM department to do their reviews.

Sometimes, clinical personnel obtain control of the record postdischarge in order to complete their documentation. While this activity is certainly laudable and ultimately facilitates processing, it causes delay in HIM processing and increases the risk of the chart being lost or damaged. Further, removing the chart from normal processing also removes it from the oversight of other clinical or administrative personnel, thereby providing an opportunity for an individual to tamper with the record, if he or she were so motivated. However unlikely this scenario may seem, it serves to remind the reader that the medical record is a legal document and, in a court of law, is admissible as evidence under the revised Business Record Rule (Federal Rules of Evidence 2014).

Therefore, every effort must be made to ensure that processing proceeds as prescribed in the HIM department's policies and procedures manual, which addresses necessary state and federal regulation that directly impact the HIM department's daily operations. HIM personnel who are responsible for obtaining control of the discharged records must be guided by clear procedures to identify and follow-up on records whose location has not been identified on a timely basis.

Finally, the record may be routed to another clinical area for continuing patient care. For example, a patient is readmitted two days after discharge and the physician has requested the prior record to be reviewed on the nursing unit. If this record is transmitted before processing, there is a danger of the old record being commingled with the new admission or pages might be lost. HIM should always bind such records into a folder to minimize these risks. If possible, without delaying patient care, the record should at least be coded before it is sent to the clinical area.

In an EHR environment, test results, dictations, and other types of documentation are available to clinicians and reviewers, and it may not be necessary to provide immediate access to residual paper. However, in the hybrid record environment, policies and procedures for access to records in process must be observed.

Impact of Clinical Documentation Improvement

As discussed in chapter 5, clinical documentation improvement (CDI) is designed to improve communication, and CDI activities can have a direct impact on postdischarge processing because, at least theoretically, any deficiencies in the documentation of care by the physician have already been identified and may have been resolved through the concurrent query process. While this impact pertains more to the coding staff than the chart completion analysts, the activity of completing the chart for other purposes may indirectly benefit the quantitative analysis process as physicians notice deficiencies on their own. Further, it is likely that a CDI specialist who notices a missing history and physical (H&P) may call this deficiency to the attention of the physician so that documentation is completed sooner rather than later.

Check Your Understanding 6.1.

1. What impact does an EHR have on timely chart completion?

2. What is the primary cause of coding backlog due to incomplete charts?

3. What is the ultimate goal of the physician query process?

Creating a Clean Claim

In general, charge capture occurs before patient discharge, and the HIM department usually does not actually enter charges. However, the HIM department may have such responsibilities in situations in which emergency department (ED) coding of visit levels is entered as charges rather than soft coding, or possibly when high-cost supply charges are entered. These situations are rare; it is more likely that HIM personnel would encounter the charge system through employment in ancillary departments, such as radiology, or in ambulatory surgery or clinic settings. In general, the post and review of charges takes place in the originating area and patient accounting, respectively. However, HIM is often in the position of having to correct errors that are related to coding.

Charge Review

Although the HIM department is not traditionally associated with charge capture, it can become involved in reviewing and analyzing charges to ensure that coding is complete or to assist in clearing failed claims. For example, a coder may review a claim that fails because a charge is missing a Current Procedural Terminology (CPT) modifier and determine which modifier is needed. This situation often occurs when there are multiple services rendered in the ED that require analysis to determine whether a modifier or different code is needed. The revenue cycle team should be provided a summary of failed claims so that processes can be reviewed and amended as needed in order to prevent such errors. An extensive discussion of claims processing is found in chapter 7.

Late Charges

The main reason for establishing a bill hold is to allow complete or clean processing of an account before the claim is filed with the payer. The two most common processing delays are coding and charging. If a chart has not been coded, the bill will not drop. However, a bill may drop if it is missing charges. For example, a patient has an ultrasound of her breast after the findings on a mammogram are abnormal. An outpatient radiology account with one charge for a mammogram will drop at the end of the bill hold because the system would have no way of knowing that abnormal findings on the x-ray prompted the physician to order an ultrasound. If the bill for the x-ray drops and transmits to the payer without the ultrasound charge, the ultrasound charge must be entered at a later date and the account will have to be rebilled. In addition, the medical necessity diagnosis for the ultrasound (usually an abnormal mammogram finding) will need to be added to the claim.

Late charges—any charges posted after the day of service—are normal and not in themselves cause for concern. After all, the purpose of the bill hold is to allow for the posting of all charges before the bill drops. However, the posting of late charges *after* the bill drops is problematic, and the reasons for the late posting should be investigated and corrected. Sometimes, tardy posting of charges is the result of unexpected volume or delays in procedures. Hourly staff who are not authorized to work overtime may defer the administrative task of charge posting to the next day. Delays such as these can be accommodated within the bill-hold period. However, departments that are chronically understaffed or that have personnel who are disorganized or inadequately trained may find themselves discovering missing charges that have to be posted long after the encounter. Some departments record their activities in their own computer systems, which then posts charges to the facility's billing system in batches during daily processing. Without daily reconciliation of these systems, those departments may not discover posting errors until after the bill has dropped.

Rebilling can diminish revenue. When late charges occur after the claim has been processed and paid, the cost of rebilling a claim may exceed the reimbursement for the missing charge. Furthermore, rebilling is tracked by payers, including CMS contractors, for potential billing-compliance problems.

Table 6.1 shows the difference in the processing of a clean claim versus one with a late charge. In this simplified example, with no additional processes involved, the cost of processing the claim literally doubles, since every step is performed twice. The cost rises dramatically when the late charge is an error or when the payer requests documentation. Therefore, minimizing late charges is a key process improvement for revenue cycle enhancement.

Revenue Code

Revenue codes identify the location of a service and are attached to the relevant charges in the charge description master (CDM). Revenue codes flow over to the uniform bill along with the procedure codes (if applicable) and the quantity and dollar amount of the charge. If a Healthcare Common Procedure Coding System (HCPCS) code must be soft coded after charging, care must be taken to ensure that the HCPCS code is appropriate to the revenue code. For example, a laboratory CPT code in the 80000 range should not be assigned to a radiology revenue code. Errors of this nature are generally chargemaster set-up or maintenance errors. To avoid these errors,

Table 6.1. The impact of late charges on process flow

Clean Claim	Late Charge with Rebilling
1. Post charges.	1. Post charges.
2. Drop bill.	2. Drop bill.
3. Review UB.	3. Review UB.
4. Transmit claim.	4. Transmit claim.
5. Receive reimbursement.	5. Receive reimbursement.
6. Post payment to account.	6. Post payment to account.
	7. Post late charge.
	8. Drop bill.
	9. Bill holds for late charge review.
	10. Query department for validity of charge.
	11. Correct the claim.
	12. Flag UB for revised claim.
	13. Transmit claim.
	14. Receive adjusted reimbursement.
	15. Post payment to account.

all changes to the chargemaster should be approved and monitored through a central department or committee. All chargemaster changes should be reviewed immediately after entering to ensure accurate data. Note that revenue codes apply only to hospitals; they are not applicable to physician-office billing.

Modifiers

For outpatient claims, Medicare requires the use of CPT/HCPCS code modifiers in certain circumstances. Modifiers communicate important information to the Medicare administrative contractor (MAC) that facilitates claims processing and calculation of reimbursement. For example, some CPT surgical codes, such as for cataract removal, are inherently unilateral. If the procedure is performed bilaterally, the modifier 50 communicates this to the MAC. Additional modifiers that enrich the data include LT/RT (left/right) and EA/EB/EC, which are applied to certain anti-anemia drug administration charges to indicate whether the patient is anemic due to chemotherapy (EA), radiation (EB), or both (EC). Modifiers are listed and explained in CPT and HCPCS code books as well as on payer websites.

Lack of appropriate modifiers could cause the bill to fail. The HIM department coding policies and procedures should include proper use of modifiers applying to outpatient cases such as those in ambulatory surgery and the ED. If the HIM department is also responsible for coding outpatient clinic records, such policies and procedures will be extremely important.

Data Validation

Throughout the facility, data are collected and entered into the computer system. A small ED with only 50 visits per day generates approximately 1,500 visits a month. At an average price of $3,000 per visit, the monthly gross revenue is around $4.5 million. Even with an accuracy rate of 99 percent, 15 of these records ($45,000) will not bill on a timely basis. Looking at the volume of data that is collected for each patient, potentially hundreds of fields will be in error and require correction, holding up billing and slowing cash flow. Even using a subcategory on a reason-for-visit code (for example, using only the first five digits of a six-digit ICD-10-CM code) prevents a clean claim. For this reason alone, computer data-validation edits are essential front-end tools. The need for data validation applies to all aspects of data collection—not just financial applications.

Even when data collection is 100 percent accurate, there are still occasions when patient data must be changed to reflect a change in circumstance. For example, a newborn may be listed in the system as baby boy Jones when discharged home, but when he comes to the ED 15 days after discharge, he is named Joe Jones. The name on the medical record will need to be updated. Some issues requiring correction are identified in the HIM department, others are also corrected there. Depending on the facility's needs and the way the systems are designed, routing of data corrections might be to a central data quality area or might be the responsibility of the originating department. Whatever the process, there need to be policies and procedures in place to ensure that data correction is done promptly, accurately, and with an informative audit trail.

The need for an audit trail is two-fold. First, any change to patient data needs to be documented. Patient records are discoverable for legal purposes, and any and all changes to that record must be identified. Second, it is important that changes be made only for legitimate purposes. Therefore, an audit trail is an important internal control mechanism to ensure that all changes are verifiable with the author of that change. One way to analyze the audit trail is to document trends in changes to determine whether certain changes or occurrences are happening in a particular area or by one particular person. Concomitant with the need for an audit trail is a facility-wide procedure to ensure that access to change data is limited to only those individuals with the appropriate authority to make the change.

From the HIM perspective, coders need to be able to change codes if they have made an error. They also need to be able to add modifiers where appropriate, and they need access to amend some errors in data, such as discharge disposition. Occasionally, other errors such as the incorrect entry of a patient's gender are noted and coders may be permitted to correct this field as well. The fields that HIM personnel are permitted to amend should be listed in the HIM department's policies and procedures manual. It is unlikely that personnel other than coders would have occasion to make such changes, and access to files should therefore be limited to read-only in those cases.

As mentioned in chapter 4, errors in assignment of medical record numbers can result in a patient being assigned more than one number. In these cases, the HIM department is typically responsible for analyzing the records, determining what correction needs to be made, and ultimately merging the records as needed. Although this error is typically attributed to patient access, it is not always avoidable. Computer down time may result in duplicate medical record number assignments, and patient name changes (such as giving a nickname on the first visit but a full first name on subsequent visits) sometimes make finding prior records difficult. Of course, deliberate subterfuge on the part of the patient is occasionally the root cause.

Although merging health records may not seem like a revenue cycle issue, bear in mind that patient accounts are grouped by health record number. For example, Richard Wilson visits the hospital for laboratory tests in conjunction with an annual physical exam. The next day, Wilson collapses in the grocery store and is rushed to the ED of the same hospital. He is subsequently admitted for treatment of an acute myocardial infarction. Wilson does not have his wallet with him in the ambulance, and he is registered in the ED as Dick Wilson, the name his wife gives the emergency medical technicians at the grocery store. This patient now has two medical record numbers and one account under each. For most payers, this issue can be addressed at some point in the future with no problem. However, if Mr. Wilson is a Medicare patient, the CMS three-day payment window requires that the laboratory account and the inpatient account must be combined for billing purposes. Because the accounts are under two different medical record numbers, most computer systems will not detect the potential account combination.

Although this is an extreme example, it highlights the potential revenue cycle implications of seemingly mundane issues like medical record number assignment. A quick sort of the DNFB will yield potential duplicates, and records with similar last names should be reviewed for this issue. The HIM department routinely conducts audits of the master patient index; however, this activity is likely not timely for billing purposes.

Patient Status and Disposition Changes

Another unavoidable type of change involves a patient who enters the facility as an outpatient and is subsequently admitted as an inpatient. Since the coding and billing requirements, not to mention the documentation requirements, of inpatients and outpatients are very different, the patient's registration data will have to be amended. This change cannot wait until after discharge because automatic charges such as accommodations are driven by patient type and room type. For example, an ED patient who is admitted to the intensive care unit (ICU) but left as an ED patient in the computer system will not receive ICU room charges. If the patient type is changed in the middle of the stay, the bill will fail for missing room charges between the admission date and the type change date. The documentation must then be analyzed to determine exactly when the patient was admitted, and the charges and admission date would need to be adjusted accordingly.

Policies and procedures must be in place to ensure that patient access is notified immediately of any change in the patient's location so that the system can be updated promptly. Occasionally, errors are made in interpreting the physician's order to admit. For example, the order states admit to observation—an outpatient status—but the person taking the order incorrectly enters an order to admit and the patient is assigned inpatient status. Sometimes, this type of error is not caught until after discharge. Therefore, HIM personnel—coders and analysts—should be alert to the wording of admission orders and should bring any potential problems to the attention of case management and patient access immediately so that the case can be evaluated and errors in registration and automatic charges can be corrected before billing.

It is the opinion of this author that changes in patient-type data should be the responsibility of one centralized unit. The access to change this type of data, particularly postdischarge, should be limited to a few highly trained individuals who are authorized to make the change and knowledgeable about the additional issues that must be addressed, such as room charges and bill type. Although assignment of this task to patient accounting is certainly a legitimate choice, it also makes sense to house the task in patient access, where concurrent changes should have been made in the first place. Assigning the task to patient access simplifies communication and enables patient access to focus on process improvement.

Two additional issues of note are related changes to the patient's discharge data: the timely documentation of a discharge log and accurate discharge-status reporting. Once the physician writes a discharge order, it is up to the nursing staff to get the patient out of the facility and to record the time and date of that event. If staff are busy, the task of logging out the patient may not take place concurrently with the event and, if done hours later, may overlap the patient's admission to another facility, such as skilled nursing. Similarly, if the discharge disposition is *home* but the patient actually was transferred to another facility, there may be reimbursement implications.

Members of the patient access department will notice delayed discharging if they see that beds are routinely open at the same time every afternoon. HIM coders may also notice data showing that outpatients are admitted and discharged at exactly the same time on the same day. Accurate timing of admission and discharge may impact the validity of subsequent audit reviews, so anomalies in these data should be reported back to the clinical departments for education and correction.

HIM coders should validate the discharge disposition of all records that they code. For example, reimbursement-sharing issues arise in transfers to long-term care hospitals (LTCHs), and payers will note patients whose discharge status does not match subsequent care. Additionally, if a Medicare patient is transferred from one inpatient prospective payment system (IPPS) hospital to another, CMS states that "Payment is made to the final discharging hospital at the full prospective payment rate. Payment to the transferring hospital is based upon a per diem rate (that is, the prospective payment rate divided by the average length of stay for the specific DRG [diagnosis-related group] into which the case falls and multiplied by the patient's length of stay at the transferring hospital)" (CMS 2014). Failure to report the correct discharge disposition on a claim is considered a claim error and may result in payment for the claim being denied. CMS publication 100-04, Medicare Claims Processing, details billing rules. It is available in the Internet-Only Manuals (IOM) section of the CMS website (CMS 2008–2015).

Check Your Understanding 6.2.

1. What is a late charge and why is it important?

2. Why is prebilling data validation important?

3. Describe a problem that can occur if patient status is not accurate during the patient's visit.

Monitoring Coding Quality

Even the most experienced coders make occasional errors. With an accuracy rate of 97 percent, 3 out of every 100 charts contains an error. In the inpatient setting, errors that affect the DRGs are particularly problematic. Even payers that do not reimburse on DRGs often use DRGs for evaluating medical necessity, establishing per diem or per procedure rates, and tracking quality of care. Therefore, coding accuracy is important regardless of the payer. For payers that reimburse on DRGs, coding accuracy is critical. In the outpatient setting, the matching of diagnosis and procedure codes with accurate modifiers, as needed, is essential. Providers should not wait for denials to tell them that there is a coding quality issue. Instead, the following stages of coding review should take place routinely:

- Prebilling review
- Targeted review (for example, specific DRGs, claims with no comorbidity/complication (CC) or major comorbidity/complication (MCC), claims with certain CCs or MCCs, medical necessity for certain procedures)
- Random reviews for accuracy benchmarks

Prebilling Reviews

Ideally, every record should be reviewed before billing for coding accuracy, particularly pertaining to the diagnoses that drive DRG assignment and completeness of the coding of procedures. Because such a process would require nearly double the usual coding staff, a review of every record before billing rarely happens. However, the volume of prebilling reviews can be reduced by a few factors to make the task manageable for most facilities. Prebilling review must be done within the bill-hold period, so speed is essential. Data analysis is helpful to reduce the volume of reviews.

To begin data analysis, obtain a report containing the coded data for all patients discharged on the day under review. Some systems have standard reports for this type of data; others may have existing reports that incidentally contain the data. For example, a physician index for the day is just as useful as a disease index, as long as the physician index lists diagnosis and procedure codes. If the report can be obtained electronically, that is best because the data can then be sorted by principal diagnosis (or DRG) for efficiency. Ideally, the report should also contain the charges for the account. If not, obtain the detailed DNFB and sort it by descending dollar value. If this type of report cannot easily be obtained, use the coding summary or attestation sheets that are usually available when the coding is finalized.

The type and detail of review performed on a daily basis will depend on the coding staff and the historical error patterns. At a minimum, look at all charts that contain issues previously identified on coding audits. Pay attention to known issues that are the subject of scrutiny from the Office of Inspector General (OIG) and recovery audit contractor (RAC) as well as issues that appear on comprehensive error-rate testing (CERT) reports. (Refer to chapter 7 for a list of agencies to consider when developing a coding monitoring plan.) Web addresses for the current plans and focus can be found in the resources list at the end of this chapter. Keep a log of charts reviewed for compliance documentation and report error rates as a performance improvement project using random audits as the baseline for improvement. For outpatient records, make sure every account contains a visit-level code and that essential modifiers are present. For surgery cases, ensure that all cases contain procedure codes or the appropriate procedure-cancellation code. Once a process has been developed and implemented, daily review of charts can be done in a reasonable amount of time.

Targeted Reviews

Targeted reviews, such as diagnosis-specific reviews, are useful to determine whether a known error has been repeated by one or more coders or whether documentation improvement is needed. For DRG-based payers, targeted reviews are particularly important. Coding managers should continue to review any issue that arises from an audit until ongoing correction of that issue has been made. For example, if coders tend to miss coding a peripherally inserted central catheter (PICC) line, then an audit of records with a PICC line charge can be done daily until 100 percent accuracy is maintained for a period of time.

Random Audits

Routine random audits for coding accuracy should be done, preferably by an external auditor. In the absence of funding for external audits, coders can review each other's charts. Alternatively, the coding supervisor or manager can allocate several hours a week for the purpose of random audits. Only random audits can be extrapolated to express overall accuracy rates. Further, it is the opinion of this author that only all-payer, all-patient audits provide a true picture of an individual coder's accuracy. Figure 6.1 shows the steps for selecting random cases for audit.

Figure 6.1. Selecting cases for random audit

1. Obtain a list of all cases for the period.
2. Select a sample size, based on the goals of the audit.
   Example: 10% of 2,000 discharges = Sample size of 200 cases
3. Sort the cases by discharge date or in another systematic order, such as account number.
4. Number the cases.
5. Obtain a list of random numbers that is at least as long as the sample size. Random.org, listed in Resources at the end of this chapter, is a good source for randomized numbers.
6. Based on the number of digits in the random number list, decide how many and which digits of the random number will be used and determine how to handle numbers that are larger than the total list of cases.
7. Select a starting point in the random number list.
8. Beginning with the starting point, for each number on the random list, find and mark the number of the case with that number.
9. Continue matching until the sample size is reached.

With a random audit, meaningful error rates can be calculated. Typically, error rates are calculated two ways: the number of records in which there is an error as a percentage of the total number of records reviewed, and the number of code selection errors by category as a percentage of the total number of correct codes assigned. These main categories can then be broken out, for example, by coder, DRG, diagnosis, or procedure. It is particularly useful to categorize errors by the type of error, such as error in selecting the principal diagnosis, error in selecting the CPT/HCPCS modifier, and error in optimizing the DRG. Drilling down in this manner helps frame objectives for coder remediation as well as future targeted audits.

Internal and External Auditing Processes

The importance of quality monitoring cannot be overemphasized. Because coded data is used for billing, case-mix analysis, and other critical purposes, every effort must be made to ensure that it is accurate and timely. Both the coding and the resultant data entry must be routinely scrutinized because a coder might select a correct code but enter it incorrectly. Quality monitoring is typically achieved through an audit process.

Internal Audits

Best practice for internal auditing is to review all Medicare and other DRG-based payer records prior to billing. If staffing issues prevent a review of all records, target audits of problem issues should be conducted.

For the purpose of revenue cycle management, it is preferable to audit the records before billing. With a short bill-hold period, prebilling audits may not be possible or practical. In that case, every effort should be made to audit the records within the payer's rebilling period (discussed in chapter 7).

One way to handle prebilling reviews is to target specific diagnoses or DRGs that have been identified as problematic on past audits. A list of such diagnoses should be developed from historical audits, and each facility's list will be different. Some diagnoses should always be reviewed, such as chest pain, congestive heart failure, and sepsis. For example, chest pain is a symptom, and documentation could be reviewed to determine whether a more definitive diagnosis could be obtained. A list of high-risk DRGs relative to recovery audit contractor (RAC) audits should also be reviewed on a regular basis. Such a list can be developed by reviewing ongoing RAC-approved issues across all regions. As these tend to mirror problematic issues already identified by OIG audits and CERT reports, there is not a great deal of controversy regarding focus.

External Audits

Because a coding team can err as a group, it is best practice to have external auditors periodically review coding quality. External audits should report error rates in multiple ways so that the facility can obtain a clear understanding of the coding education needs. For example, an error rate of 60 percent based on charts, in which all of the errors are missing minor secondary codes, does not have the same implications as an error rate of 60 percent based on the number of codes assigned, in which half are erroneous principal diagnoses that changed the DRG assignment. External auditors should report back errors by type, coder, and presumed reason. Presumed reasons can include coder error, missing documentation at the time of coding, and documentation clarity.

External audits tend to pay for themselves either by finding errors that can be rebilled for increased reimbursement or by finding overbilled accounts that can be rebilled to avoid RAC recoupment. Ultimately, routine audits help establish a pattern of compliance with coding quality standards.

Present on Admission Status

With the advent of Medicare severity diagnosis-related groups (MS-DRGs), CMS began to implement a policy of not paying for certain cases of **hospital-acquired conditions (HACs)**, which are preventable conditions that develop while the patient is hospitalized. For example, in many instances, a stage III decubitus (pressure) ulcer is a CC that bumps up reimbursement to a higher paying DRG. If the ulcer was **present on admission (POA)**, meaning that the patient had the condition coded when admitted to the hospital, CMS will pay the higher rate in consideration of the resource intensity of the case. If the ulcer was *not* POA, it is considered a HAC and CMS will disregard the ulcer code in the grouping, which may cause the case to be reimbursed at a lower rate. In response to pressure from CMS, some states have also implemented this policy for Medicaid reimbursement (CMS 2015d). Because POA status has implications for reimbursement, it should be subject to the same audit criteria as the codes themselves. The HACs that will not be paid at the higher rate include the following (CMS 2015b):

- Foreign object retained after surgery
- Air embolism
- Blood incompatibility
- Stage III and stage IV pressure ulcers
- Falls and trauma:
  - Fractures
  - Dislocations
  - Intracranial injuries
  - Crushing injuries
  - Burn
  - Other injuries
- Manifestations of poor glycemic control
  - Diabetic ketoacidosis
  - Nonketotic hyperosmolar coma
  - Hypoglycemic coma
  - Secondary diabetes with ketoacidosis
  - Secondary diabetes with hyperosmolarity
- Catheter-associated urinary tract infection (UTI)
- Vascular catheter-associated infection
- Surgical site infection, mediastinitis, following coronary artery bypass graft (CABG)
- Surgical site infection following bariatric surgery for obesity
  - Laparoscopic gastric bypass
  - Gastroenterostomy
  - Laparoscopic gastric restrictive surgery
- Surgical site infection following certain orthopedic procedures
  - Spine
  - Neck
  - Shoulder
  - Elbow
- Surgical site infection following cardiac implantable electronic device (CIED)
- Deep vein thrombosis (DVT)/pulmonary embolism (PE) following certain orthopedic procedures
  - Total knee replacement
  - Hip replacement
- Iatrogenic pneumothorax with venous catheterization

The 14 categories of HACs listed here include the new HACs from the IPPS fiscal year (FY) 2013 final rule, which are surgical site infection following CIED and iatrogenic pneumothorax with venous catheterization. No additional HACs were added for FY 2014 or FY 2015 (CMS

2015b). The specific ICD-1-CM codes associated with HAC conditions are available on the CMS HAC website.

Case-Mix Index in MS-DRGs

In aggregate, the implementation of MS-DRGs does not change the case-mix index (CMI) calculation. However, MS-DRGs have made the analysis of changes in CMI somewhat more difficult. Under version 24 and earlier versions, most DRGs came in pairs: with CC or without CC. It was easy to see a change in the percentage of cases that fell in the lower paying (without CC) DRG versus the higher paying (with CC) DRG. With version 25, CMS began converting these pairs to three-level sets (with MCC, with CC but no MCC, and without CC or MCC), and version 26 completed the transition. Without a history of how a facility's cases fall into these three levels, it became difficult to determine whether changes in CMI came from coding issues or real changes in practice patterns or severity. Obtaining an understanding of this issue often requires the assistance of consultants.

If the facility has the ability to regroup cases from prior years into the current three-level MS-DRG version, some historical perspective can be obtained. From FY 2008 forward, most of the DRGs are in sets and can be compared on a relatively level playing field. Table 6.2 illustrates the benefit of reviewing FY 2015 MS-DRGs in sets. (The FY 2015 MS-DRGs are listed in the online resources that accompany this book.) Viewing the data in sets helps to construct targeted audits and identify potential coding issues. For example, organizing historical data in sets, variances in case mix within the set can help the facility see whether there have been significant changes in the mix between cases with and without CC and MCC. Significant changes should be reviewed for possible coding or documentation issues. In table 6.2, for example, the volume of cases with and without MCC is inverted in 2014 and 2015, compared to 2013. Continuous monitoring of such changes enables coding managers to correct errors in a timely basis and provides administrators with valuable information about case mix.

Impact of Internal Guidelines

The development of internal guidelines for coding quality is facility-specific and depends on the centralization or decentralization of the coding function. Nevertheless, all areas that are responsible for coding must have policies and procedures in place to ensure consistent, accurate coding of cases.

Establishing Standards

The foundations for coding policies and procedures are the *ICD-10-CM Official Guidelines for Coding and Reporting* and *ICD-10-PCS Official Guidelines for Coding and Reporting* (HHS 2015a, HHS 2015b). Building on those guidelines are *Coding Clinic* and *CPT Assistant*. Beyond the strict application of these guidelines, Medicare and Medicaid rules should also be considered. For example, coder responsibility for data quality should extend to review of the patient account data for Medicare code edits (CMS 2015c). Additional coding guidelines at the facility level can

Table 6.2. Sample three-year comparison of signs-and-symptoms case volume with and without major comorbidities and complications (MCCs)

MS-DRG	MS-DRG Title	Annual Number of Cases		
		2013	2014	2015
947	Signs and symptoms with MCC	36	2	5
948	Signs and symptoms without MCC	5	23	70

be developed as described in chapter 1 of *Effective Management of Coding Services* (Gentul and Davis 2011), an excerpt of which is included in online appendix 6.1. The following section on orientation process is adapted from the same source.

Orientation Process

Many, if not most, healthcare facilities have a regularly scheduled 1- or 2-day orientation program for all new employees, regardless of job function. The purpose of the orientation program is to introduce new employees to the following:

- Organization as a whole
- Department in which he or she will work
- Specific job responsibilities

Depending on facility policy, new employees may be required to attend an orientation to the overall organization before attending their department-specific orientation. Therefore, their start date is not necessarily the date they actually begin to produce work. As a practical matter, coding managers should assume that the new employee's first week is devoted primarily to orientation. Orientation to the overall organization might include discussion of the following:

- Confidentiality
- Joint Commission requirements
- Occupational Safety and Health Administration (OSHA) requirements
- Issues related to the Health Insurance Portability and Accountability Act (HIPAA)
- Corporate compliance plan
- State requirements
- Employee benefits
- Expectations of conduct

When possible, orientation topics should be presented in order of importance. For example, the facility's confidentiality policies should be presented before the location of the cafeteria is discussed. Typically, the human resources (HR) department conducts the orientation to the organization, with support from other departments. For instance, the privacy officer may be asked to present the topic of confidentiality to new employees. Certainly one purpose of this process is to impart the tone and culture of the organization. However, the orientation also gives new employees the opportunity to ask questions they may have thought of since accepting employment. It is important that new employees receive accurate answers to their questions. Orientation, therefore, should be conducted by experienced individuals who can provide answers themselves or query others effectively to obtain prompt answers.

The new employee's workstation should be ready upon his or her arrival. Orientation to the department should begin after he or she has settled in. Introductions should be the first order of business and can be made during an informal tour of the department.

The coding manager or designee overseeing the orientation to the department should have a checklist of items to be discussed and information to be disseminated. (See figure 6.2 for a sample orientation checklist.) The facility may use a generic form with space included for departmental specifics. Current Joint Commission standards can be used to ensure that the checklist includes all the requirements of continued employment, such as verification that the employee has read and understood the organizational mission statement and confidentiality policy.

The policies and procedures manual and the HIM department's table of organization also should be reviewed and discussed. Sections that do not necessarily pertain to the employee's immediate job function may be covered to provide an overall picture of the department's functions and responsibilities. The department also may have the new staff member rotate through all or most of the job functions. Actually seeing the functions in action helps to clarify the department's role within the healthcare facility.

The new employee should sign off on the checklist to indicate that the orientation process has been completed. The checklist then should be signed and dated by the HIM manager or a supervisor. It may be kept in the HR department or in the employee's file within the HIM department. In addition, a confidentiality statement should be signed with the signature witnessed and dated. The confidentiality statement then should be reviewed annually or according to organizational policy. Any employee-specific confidential information, such as computer passwords, must be kept in a secure location.

The next part of the new employee's orientation is to address the specific functions of the job. To be fully functional in, and comfortable with, the new position, the new coder first must be instructed on the department's operations. For example, the following topics may be addressed:

- How is work distributed?
- What tasks are to be performed in addition to coding?
- What happens to the health record after it is coded?

These and other functional orientations are listed in figure 6.2. One important reason for formalizing this review is to document that it occurred. This documentation ensures that a lack of knowledge of job functions cannot be used as an excuse for incomplete work. Orientation to the functions of the job also should do the following:

- Review the regulatory requirements that affect the position
- Determine the need for training
- Clarify the standards used to measure the employee's progress
- Explain the probationary period
- Discuss the job productivity expectations

Regulatory Requirements

Healthcare facilities and their employees must meet numerous regulatory and accreditation standards. The coding manager should review the facility's corporate compliance, coding compliance, and performance-improvement programs with the new coder.

Often, the arrival of a new employee gives the HIM department the opportunity to involve the entire coding staff in a formal review of the facility's regulatory and compliance programs. Although this sort of review is typically an annual education process throughout the organization, drawing the existing staff into a new coder's training process is helpful for reinforcement.

In addition to the above training, employees must receive role-based training on meaningful use (MU). Although it is not necessarily relevant for staff to understand all the nuances of the program, they should be knowledgeable about their role in ensuring the successful implementation and maintenance of their part in the MU compliance process. For example, release-of-information staff must functionally implement electronic release of information (ROI) requirements. Therefore, they must understand what is required and how to comply.

Coding Quality and Training

A new employee's need for training can be based on the areas of weakness identified from the coding test taken during the interviewing process. The coding manager should schedule education and training in these areas before the coder begins the actual work of coding. Ongoing quality reviews and education should be provided as a part of the continuing education process

Figure 6.2. Functional orientation

Functional Orientation

EMPLOYEE NAME: _____

Hire Date: _____ Orientation Completion Date: _____

DATE	DESCRIPTION	Supervisor Initials	Employee Initials
	Tour of the department		
	Tour of departments relevant to function (list)		
	Orientation to system modules		
	Orientation to policies and procedures		
	Work distribution process		
	Ancillary tasks to be performed		
	Work completion process		
	Supervisory process		
	Productivity requirements and reporting		
	Email/Internet use		
	Work environment responsibilities		
	Copy of performance evaluation criteria provided and discussed, including probationary period		
	Immediate training needs (list)		

for all coding professionals. Training duration depends on the experience level of the coder. Sometimes, the focus of training is orientation to the EHR. However, if an inexperienced coder is being trained, formal education and continuous monitoring may be necessary. The duration of training, then, is reflective of the amount and type of material being conveyed as well as the speed with which the trainee absorbs it. Training is an ongoing process. While initial training gets a coding professional up to speed in the department, ongoing training is needed as coding professionals progress from the beginning level to higher levels, such as from coding ancillary accounts to coding inpatient cases.

The coding manager should discuss all identified coding errors with new employees. Occasionally, the reviewer is wrong. Unless the error is clear, new employees should be given the opportunity to defend their coding with authoritative references. This process enables them to develop a collaborative relationship with the coding supervisor and their coworkers that will have long-term benefits.

Standards of Measurement

One goal of the functional orientation is to ensure that the new coder understands the standards that will be used to measure his or her job performance. For example, the following questions may be addressed:

- How often is performance reviewed?
- Who performs the review?
- How will errors be handled?

All employees should be given routine, collaborative, and educational feedback. This feedback is particularly important for new coders, who find it unproductive and stressful to wonder for weeks or months how well they are doing.

Probationary Period

An employee hired to fill an open position generally serves a period of probation. The intent of the **probationary period** is to give the employee the opportunity to demonstrate his or her ability to perform the duties of the position.

Most states specify the duration of the probationary period, which typically is three months. The probationary period is the last opportunity the employer has to rectify a hiring error with minimal effort. Probationary periods typically can be extended at weekly or monthly intervals, but usually last no more than six months.

If the new employee's work during the probationary period is unsatisfactory, the coding manager should identify the specific areas that need improvement and then discuss possible remedies with the probationary coder. Ideally, the new employee will demonstrate steady progress throughout this period. When the new employee has progressed, even though not meeting every expectation, the coding manager must decide whether to extend the probationary period or remove the coder from probationary status.

During the probationary period, healthcare facilities often compensate an employee at less than full pay and withhold certain benefits, such as health insurance. The purpose of the probationary period is to ensure that the potential coder is qualified for the position, not to "buy time" to interview other candidates. The coding manager should not "string along" an individual for an extended period of time without making a decision. Organizations that engage in such unfair and unethical hiring practices will soon become known in the coding community and begin to experience hiring difficulties.

Terminating an employee after he or she has been taken off probation can be difficult and stressful. Thus, to avoid difficulties, the coding manager should be aware of all written policies, legalities, and union agreements regarding probationary periods and the hiring and firing of staff.

Productivity Expectations

The productivity expectations of the position should be clearly stated. An employee's failure to meet productivity standards can be grounds for dismissal. The coding manager who treats productivity expectations lightly is likely to end up with unproductive employees and will no doubt be held accountable by department management and administration as overall productivity declines.

Two measures of a coder's skill are the types of errors he or she makes and the speed at which he or she can work. For example, coders who achieve 100 percent accuracy in assigning principal diagnoses and DRG groupings but occasionally miss an additional diagnosis are more accurate than those who make mistakes selecting principal diagnoses and DRGs but correctly code everything else. All coding is important, but correct coding of principal diagnoses and DRGs produces the most benefits and the least need for recoding after quality audits.

However, the coder who completes only one health record per day with 100 percent accuracy is clearly not productive. The speed at which a coder can work depends on a number of factors, including the quality of the documentation in the health record and the extent of his or her responsibilities as well as the service line. Typically, inpatient coders complete fewer records per day than outpatient coders. Coders can also code more health records in a day when they do not also have to abstract and enter data. On the other hand, coders who enter their own data have the opportunity to review the results and correct errors at the time of entry. Computer-assisted coding affects volume productivity, and the structure of the EHR interface can also affect coder performance. For all of these reasons, coder productivity is best considered a performance improvement activity: the department and its personnel should be always striving to improve current performance rather than attempting to achieve external benchmarks that may be unrealistic in the existing environment. That being said, it is useful to network with colleagues who have the same EHR system and coder responsibilities to determine what expectations might be realistic.

Impact of Noncoding Activities

Noncoding activities negatively affect accuracy and speed. It is important to view departmental functions as a whole. Some employees seem to attract unrelated projects, either because of their helpful personality traits or their desire for job enrichment or because they want to demonstrate supervisory capabilities. Therefore, supervisory personnel should monitor employee activities to ensure that work distribution and workflow are appropriate.

Check Your Understanding 6.3.

1. List three stages of coding quality review.

2. What is the purpose of a random audit of coded data?

3. What is the importance of present-on-admission status?

Special Considerations for Specific Practice Settings

Coding guidelines vary between inpatient and outpatient records, and inpatient and outpatient reimbursement methodologies are different from one another. Charge-capture issues also vary by setting. The volume of material that an inpatient coder must review before assigning a code is much greater than the volume of materials an outpatient coder uses to add the correct specificity digits to a code from a physician encounter form. Herein are issues unique to these settings.

Inpatient Settings

For inpatient visits, the integration of outpatient into inpatient accounts is a unique issue. Although this task technically applies only to Medicare cases, the potential for accounts to start out as commercial ones and end up being billed to Medicare is strong, particularly for an elderly patient. In addition, some payers follow Medicare guidelines with regard to combining outpatient and inpatient accounts. Therefore, facilities may choose to make a blanket rule that all accounts that fall into this category be combined—regardless of payer. Although this rule may result in some loss of revenue, the risk of *not* combining accounts is lessened. POA status is also unique to hospital inpatients, and facilities should be alert to the adoption of Medicare's policy by other payers, particularly Medicaid.

Outpatient Settings

For outpatient accounts, medical necessity and accurate charge capture are important issues. Although reimbursement is based on the procedures rather than the diagnosis, the latter is key in determining why the procedure was performed. Abdominal pain, for example, is not an appropriate diagnosis associated with a mammogram. A diagnosis code of Z12.31, Encounter for screening mammogram for malignant neoplasm of breast, is typically sufficient to justify a screening mammogram, but the code for abnormal mammogram findings might be needed to justify a subsequent ultrasound.

Charge capture is a key issue for several reasons. One visit may generate multiple ambulatory payment classification (APC) payments. Failure to capture all of the charges may reduce reimbursement on that basis. Also, bills will fail or be denied by the payer if multiple charges for bundled services are reported (as discussed in chapter 5). Further, some charges are not logical in the absence of other charges. For example, a charge for certain vaccines without a charge for the associated injection will cause the bill to fail.

Physician Practices

The foundation for physician-practice coding is the correct assignment of evaluation and management (E/M) codes. In general, the use of a superbill form supports physician office billing, as discussed in chapter 5. However, in recent years, there has been increased conversation about the relationship between physician billing and the associated hospital billing. For example, a hospital admission may be denied payment due to lack of medical necessity; however, the physician bills for and is paid for each visit to the patient for the denied visit. Because it was the physician's order that prompted the admission in the first place, this paradox of reimbursement is problematic. During the RAC demonstration project, some hospital recoupments prompted follow-up to the physician billing. One example is multiple cases in which excisional debridement was coded but insufficiently documented on both the hospital and the physician side. Providers should be alert to expansion of this audit strategy.

Check Your Understanding 6.4.

1. Identify two types of records that should be subject to targeted internal review.

2. List two issues unique to inpatient billing.

3. List two issues critical to outpatient billing.

References

American Health Information Management Association (AHIMA). 2013. Guidelines for achieving a compliant query practice. *Journal of AHIMA* 84(2): 50–53.

Centers for Medicare and Medicaid Services (CMS). 2015a. Conditions of Participation—Hospitals. Code of Federal Regulations, Title 42, Chapter 4, Part 482.24(C)(4)(viii). http://www.ecfr.gov/cgi-bin/text-idx?SID=7de9c3a8da3771cced64bb4b577dae8f&mc=true&node=se42.5.482_124&rgn=div8.

Centers for Medicare and Medicaid Services (CMS). 2015b. Hospital Acquired Conditions. https://www.cms.gov/Medicare/Medicare-Fee-for-Service-Payment/HospitalAcqCond/Hospital-Acquired_Conditions.html.

Centers for Medicare and Medicaid Services (CMS). 2015c. Definitions of Medicare Code Edits. FY 2016 Final Rule. https://www.cms.gov/Medicare/Medicare-Fee-for-Service-Payment/AcuteInpatientPPS/FY2016-IPPS-Final-Rule-Home-Page-Items/FY2016-IPPS-Final-Rule-Data-Files.html.

Centers for Medicare and Medicaid Services (CMS). 2014. Medicare Claims Processing Manual Chapter 3: Inpatient Hospital Billing 40.2.4—IPPS Transfers Between Hospitals, Section A. http://www.cms.hhs.gov/manuals/downloads/clm104c03.pdf.

Centers for Medicare and Medicaid Services (CMS). 2008. State Medicaid Director Letter #08-004, July 31, 2008. http://www.cms.hhs.gov/SMDL/downloads/SMD073108.pdf.

Federal Rules of Evidence. 2014. Rules of Evidence. http://www.uscourts.gov/rules-policies/current-rules-practice-procedure.

Gentul, M.K. and N. Davis. 2011. Structure and organization of the coding function. Chapter 1 in *Effective Management of Coding Services,* 4th ed. Edited by L.A. Schraffenberger and L. Kuehn. Chicago: AHIMA.

Joint Commission. 2015a. RC.01.03.01 In *Record of Care in Accreditation Program: Hospitals, Accreditation Participation Requirements.* Oakbrook Terrace, IL: Joint Commission.

Joint Commission. 2015b. RC.02.04.01 In *Record of Care in Accreditation Program: Hospitals, Accreditation Participation Requirements.* Oakbrook Terrace, IL: Joint Commission.

Joint Commission. 2015c. RC.02.01.03 In *Record of Care in Accreditation Program: Hospitals, Accreditation Participation Requirements.* Oakbrook Terrace, IL: Joint Commission.

Joint Commission. 2014. Facts about ORYX for Hospitals (National Hospital Quality Measures. http://www.jointcommission.org/AccreditationPrograms/Hospitals/ORYX/oryx_facts.htm.

US Department of Health and Human Services (HHS). 2015a. ICD-10-CM Official Guidelines for Coding and Reporting. https://www.cms.gov/Medicare/Coding/ICD10/Downloads/2016-ICD-10-CM-Guidelines.pdf.

US Department of Health and Human Services (HHS). 2015b. ICD-10-PCS Official Guidelines for Coding and Reporting. https://www.cms.gov/Medicare/Coding/ICD10/Downloads/2016-Official-ICD-10-PCS-Coding-Guidelines-.pdf.

Additional Resources

American Health Information Management Association (AHIMA) Workgroup. 2014.*Clinical Documentation Improvement Toolkit.* Chicago: AHIMA.

Centers for Medicare and Medicaid Services (CMS). 2008–2015. Medicare Claims Processing Manual. https://www.cms.gov/Regulations-and-Guidance/Guidance/Manuals/Internet-Only-Manuals-IOMs-Items/CMS018912.html?DLPage=1&DLEntries=10&DLSort=0&DLSortDir=ascending.

Centers for Medicare and Medicaid Services (CMS). 2016a. Comprehensive Error Rate Testing (CERT). https://www.cms.gov/Research-Statistics-Data-and-Systems/Monitoring-Programs/Medicare-FFS-Compliance-Programs/CERT/index.html?redirect=/cert.

Centers for Medicare and Medicaid Services (CMS). 2016b. Recovery Audit Contractor (RAC) Program. https://www.cms.gov/research-statistics-data-and-systems/monitoring-programs/medicare-ffs-compliance-programs/recovery-audit-program.

Hess, P. 2015. *Clinical Documentation Improvement: Principles and Practice.* Chicago: AHIMA.

Randomness and Integrity Services Ltd. 2016. True Random Number Service. www.random.org.

Schraffenberger, L.A. and L. Kuehn, eds. 2011. *Effective Management of Coding Services.* Chicago: AHIMA.

Shaw, P. and D. Carter. 2015. *Quality and Performance Improvement in Healthcare,* 6th ed. Chicago: AHIMA.

US Department of Health and Human Services (HHS). 2016. Office of Inspector General Work Plan Archives. http://oig.hhs.gov/reports-and-publications/archives/workplan.

Claims Management

Learning Objectives

- Illustrate the importance of a clean claim.
- Compare the types of edits that are applied to claims.
- Analyze the issues that arise when a bill is denied.
- Examine the collections process.

Key Terms

- 837i
- Medically unlikely edit (MUE)
- National Correct Coding Initiative (NCCI)
- Recoupment
- Recovery audit contractor (RAC)
- Remittance advice (RA)

In a perfect patient-accounting world, reimbursement claims would drop with zero errors, transmit directly to the payer without human intervention, and be reimbursed at exactly the correct, expected amount, with all patient accounts automatically credited as soon as funds were deposited to the facility's bank account. This perfect world is not as far-fetched as it might seem.

Clean Claims

With the cooperation of all parties concerned, clean claims can be the norm. If the appropriate internal controls are in place and working, the clean claim rate can approach 100 percent. The vast preponderance of claim errors is entirely preventable. This section discusses what happens to a claim after the bill drops.

Electronic Billing

Once the bill-hold period has passed and the health information management (HIM) department has released the accounts from the hold list, uniform bill (UB) data from those accounts are compiled into an electronic transmittal file called an 837i. (Refer to figure 7.1 for UB data.) Similarly, electronic physician data are compiled into an 837p. Refer to figure 3.3 in chapter 3 for a sample CMS 1500, the paper version of the physician bill. The 837 files are formatted specifically to flag and report data in a defined format. All users who recognize this format can accept the

Figure 7.1. Uniform bill data

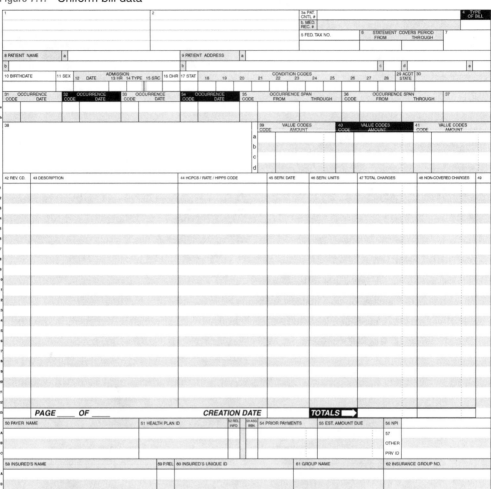

data for use in whatever function is necessary. For example, this format can be used for reporting discharge data sets to state entities as well as for reimbursement purposes.

The 837i file is transmitted to a data clearinghouse, which holds the data until they are released by the facility. While the data are being held by the clearinghouse, the facility has the opportunity to review the data to identify and correct any errors. This review is called *scrubbing the claim*, and a computer program designed to do the review is called a *scrubber*. The daily clean-claims reports from the scrubber allow a facility to see what percentage of their claims are clean on the first try and which ones are successfully billed to the payers. In the authors' experience, facilities may reasonably expect 92 percent or more of the claims to be clean the first time through the scrubber. If a sufficient level of success is not achieved, the revenue cycle departments will use the daily clean-claims reports to identify the responsible staff members and educate them on the errors so that they are not repeated.

The process of scrubbing and reviewing is an iterative one. While individual errors are certainly corrected so that specific claims can be processed, the monitoring of repetitive errors or multiple errors by specific departments or individuals is used to identify trends and opportunities for process improvement. As discussed in chapter 1, rework is wasteful. Therefore, determining the root cause of errors enables the provider to take corrective action. As frequent errors are corrected, the clean-claims rate should rise. So, the iteration of scrub, identify the cause of errors, and correct the cause eventually moves the clean-claims rate closer to 100 percent.

Providers can send claims directly to the payer without going through a clearinghouse. With paper claims, direct transmittal was the norm. With electronic claims, the proliferation of billing software combined with the unique demands of individual payers make direct relationships between the provider and its payers difficult and time consuming. With a clearinghouse, the provider makes one connection with the clearinghouse and the clearinghouse takes care of the individual payers' requirements.

The federal government contracts with a fiscal intermediary (FI) or carrier for physician service, which operates as the claims processor for Medicare. Historically, there have been 25 FIs in the United States who were dispersed by Medicare region. The Medicare contracting reform section (911) of the Medicare Prescription Drug, Improvement, and Modernization Act (2003) required Centers for Medicare and Medicaid (CMS) to replace the current FIs and carriers with new Medicare administrative contractors (MACs) in 2011 (CMS 2002). Based on this regulation change, Medicare began to combine the FI and carrier claims processing functions in each region, which resulted in the MACs providers deal with today. The new MACs, shown in table 7.1, provide beneficiary and provider service, provider enrollment, reimbursement, and payment safeguards; handle appeals; and perform provider education and training, as well as financial management, and information security.

Payment Cycle

Once a provider's claim is received by the payer, it is paid, adjusted and paid, or denied either in full or in part. If the claim is only paid partially, the payer will explain the reason for partial payment or denial within its denial code, just as it gives a reason code with explanation when a claim is denied in full.

Payment is accompanied by a transmittal explaining the relationship of the payment to the claim, which is also referred to as an explanation of benefits (EOB) or explanation of payment (EOP). Many different claims may be included in one payment, so the EOB or EOP is extremely important in order for the payer to post the cash and determine whether the payment is correct. Providers are required to have billing systems that have the capability to receive an 835 electronic-remittance advice file that is transmitted from the payer to the data clearinghouse and back into the patient accounting system, which will automatically post the file to the patients' accounts. Patient financial services (PFS) staff then reviews the accounts in the billing system to accept the electronic posting. Time is saved when the PFS staff does not have to manually post the payments to the accounts. Electronic posting also allows for tighter internal controls on the hospital's cash because payments from both the payers and patients go directly to a lockbox to be cashed. The only paperwork sent to the PFS team to process is that which is necessary to explain the claim, such as the EOB/EOP.

The patient account may be need to be adjusted to reflect allowances for contractual agreements between payers and providers. These adjustments are generally done electronically by a contract- or reimbursement-management system programmed with the hospital's managed care agreement rates and Medicare and Medicaid rates. When final bills for accounts are sent to the clearinghouse, a contractual allowance is electronically added to the account, leaving only the

Table 7.1. Medicare administrative contractors (MACs) as of April 1, 2015

MAC Jurisdiction	Previous MAC Jurisdiction	Processes Part A & Part B Claims for the following states:	MAC
DME A	DME A	Connecticut, Delaware, District of Columbia, Maine, Maryland, Massachusetts, New Hampshire, New Jersey, New York, Pennsylvania, Rhode Island, Vermont	NHIC, Inc.
DME B	DME B	Illinois, Indiana, Kentucky, Michigan, Minnesota, Ohio, Wisconsin	National Government Services, Inc.
DME C	DME C	Alabama, Arkansas, Colorado, Florida, Georgia, Louisiana, Mississippi, New Mexico, North Carolina, Oklahoma, South Carolina, Tennessee, Texas, Virginia, West Virginia, Puerto Rico, U.S. Virgin Islands	CGS Administrators, LLC
DME D	DME D	Alaska, Arizona, California, Hawaii, Idaho, Iowa, Kansas, Missouri, Montana, Nebraska, Nevada, North Dakota, Oregon, South Dakota, Utah, Washington, Wyoming, American Samoa, Guam, Northern Mariana Islands	Noridian Healthcare Solutions, LLC
5	5	Iowa, Kansas, Missouri, Nebraska	Wisconsin Physicians Service Insurance Corporation
6	6	Illinois, Minnesota, Wisconsin **HH + H for the following states:** Alaska, American Samoa, Arizona, California, Guam, Hawaii, Idaho, Michigan, Minnesota, Nevada, New Jersey, New York, Northern Mariana Islands, Oregon, Puerto Rico, US Virgin Islands, Wisconsin and Washington	National Government Services, Inc.
8	8	Indiana, Michigan	Wisconsin Physicians Service Insurance Corporation
15	15	Kentucky, Ohio **HH + H for the following states:** Delaware, District of Columbia, Colorado, Iowa, Kansas, Maryland, Missouri, Montana, Nebraska, North Dakota, Pennsylvania, South Dakota, Utah, Virginia, West Virginia, and Wyoming	CGS Administrators, LLC
E	1	California, Hawaii, Nevada, American Samoa, Guam, Northern Mariana Islands	Noridian Healthcare Solutions, LLC
F	2 & 3	Alaska, Arizona, Idaho, Montana, North Dakota, Oregon, South Dakota, Utah, Washington, Wyoming	Noridian Healthcare Solutions, LLC
H	4 & 7	Arkansas, Colorado, New Mexico, Oklahoma, Texas, Louisiana, Mississippi	Novitas Solutions, Inc.

Table 7.1.   Medicare administrative contractors (MACs) as of April 1, 2015 (Continued)

J	10	Alabama, Georgia, Tennessee	Cahaba Government Benefit Administrators, LLC
K	13 & 14	Connecticut, New York, Maine, Massachusetts, New Hampshire, Rhode Island, Vermont ****HH + H for the following states:** Connecticut, Maine, Massachusetts, New Hampshire, Rhode Island, and Vermont	National Government Services, Inc.
L	12	Delaware, District of Columbia, Maryland, New Jersey, Pennsylvania (includes Part B for counties of Arlington and Fairfax in Virginia and the city of Alexandria in Virginia)	Novitas Solutions, Inc.
M	11	North Carolina, South Carolina, Virginia, West Virginia (excludes Part B for the counties of Arlington and Fairfax in Virginia and the city of Alexandria in Virginia) ****HH + H for the following states:** Alabama, Arkansas, Florida, Georgia, Illinois, Indiana, Kentucky, Louisiana, Mississippi, New Mexico, North Carolina, Ohio, Oklahoma, South Carolina, Tennessee, and Texas	Palmetto GBA, LLC
N	9	Florida, Puerto Rico, U.S. Virgin Islands	First Coast Service Options, Inc.

**Also Processes Home Health and Hospice claims
Source: Centers for Medicare and Medicaid Services 2015a.

expected reimbursement on the account as open accounts receivable (A/R). If the patient access services team has entered the patient's co-pay, co-insurance, or deductible information, then the reimbursement system will take these factors into account, further reducing the open A/R amount on the account. The electronic adjustment system is intended to ease the PFS team's task of collecting payments owed to the hospital. The system also supports auditing, which can be used to determine whether PFS staff increased adjustments on the account in addition to the amount the reimbursement system said was owed to the hospital. As part of the month-end closing process, reports from the billing system (such as a list of accounts with very small balances) can be reviewed to see whether manual adjustments were erroneously made by PFS staff. If a pattern of errors is noted, re-education to PFS staff may be required, or there may be a contract issue with the payer that needs to be pursued as a material breach.

A claim may be denied for many reasons, some of the most common of which are lack of coverage, lack of medical necessity, and billing errors. Lack of coverage issues are related to the chapter 3 discussion of precertification issues. Optimally, the provider has verified coverage through a service or by contacting the payer, determined in advance whether the services are covered, and obtained any required preauthorization from the payer. If the patient truly is not covered for the service, then the account becomes self-pay and the provider must collect reimbursement from the patient.

Lack of medical necessity denials occur when the payer only pays for services that are justified by specific medical conditions. The patient may not have the medically necessary condition, or the patient has the condition but it was not coded on the claim. Ideally, the scrubber picks up on these issues before the claim is submitted to the payer. Some denials may be overturned by sending an explanation and a copy of the medical record to the payer, whereas if the claim is denied for a billing error, the claim can potentially be corrected and resubmitted.

Rebilling

Payers do not accept unlimited numbers of claims for the same episode of care over any length of time. Specific limitations may be stated in the payer contract or policies, and providers need to be aware of those limitations so that they are fully reimbursed. Excessive rebilling may trigger increased audit activity—another reason to drop clean claims the first time.

If a patient has more than one payer, billing to the primary payer is completed before claims are submitted to the secondary payer. In this manner, duplicate payments for the same service are avoided. Medicare is commonly the primary payer, and a wrap-around or supplemental payer covers the balance. Some primary payers, such as Medicare and Blue Cross/Blue Shield (BC/BS), send the EOB directly to the secondary payer on the patient's behalf. This process can create an issue if the secondary payer requires a different Current Procedural Terminology/Healthcare Common Procedure Coding System (CPT/HCPCS) code than the one used by the primary payer. The charge description master (CDM) is programmed to correctly use the billing code required by the primary payer. Claims denied by the secondary payer will need to be reviewed by PFS for this type of technical denial.

Check Your Understanding 7.1.

1. What is the role of a Medicare administrative contractor?

2. What is the impact of contractual agreements on claims resolution?

3. What are three common reasons for claims denials?

Use of Edits

There is really no excuse these days for submitting a faulty claim. Scrubbers are common in PFS, along with interface software that allow PFS staff to review and correct errors as well as manage workflow. No longer does the patient accounting clerk have to manually review each account line by line to validate data.

In general, all patient accounts will be reviewed electronically by an editing program that contains facility-specific, payer-specific, or other edits. Edits are written specifically to ensure that claims comply with payer rules, whether they are standard edits issued by Medicare and Medicaid or custom, state-specific edits that are built into the system. Ideally, the claim is scrubbed and corrected before the final bill is dropped. However, that is not always the case, and denied claims may be the result. Trends in denied claims will then be brought to the revenue cycle team to be reviewed and custom built into the claims scrubber system.

As noted earlier, editing is required when the diagnosis does not justify the medical necessity of the service. For example, a diagnosis of "encounter for general physical exam" does not justify a blood test for vitamin D deficiency; however, a diagnosis of osteoporosis would be sufficient. This type of edit derives from Medicare's national coverage determinations (NCDs), which are interpreted and detailed by the MACs as local coverage determinations (LCDs).

In addition to Medicare edits, there are many Medicaid edits, which vary from state to state. Commercial payer requirements can also be built into the scrubber, and there are also logical edits that should be applied so that claims are not denied for technical reasons. Examples of standard edits include matching sex-specific codes with the patient's sex, verifying that age-specific codes are appropriate for the patient's age, checking HCPCS and *International Classification of Diseases, Tenth Revision, Clinical Modification (ICD-10-CM)* code validity, and matching the diagnosis codes with the documented procedures. Examples of custom edits are bundling services that always go together—such as blood transfusion and blood products, or injections and vaccines. Edits may be constructed to ensure complete charging, such as a birth chart with a phenylketonuria (PKU) test.

Facility-Specific Edits

Each computer system has its own advantages and disadvantages. Some are turnkey systems designed to be used as-is upon implementation. Others are rules-based and are customized to the individual organization. Even with a turnkey system, additional software can be purchased that allows some customization of the system.

Front-end edits, as mentioned in chapter 4, are fairly simple in a computerized environment. These preventive controls alert users that data need attention. Such controls can prevent registrars from leaving blank fields or entering invalid dates. Failure to develop and implement edits on the front end will result in the need for expensive detective and corrective controls on the back end or, ultimately, partial or complete denial of claims. Examples of facility-specific edits include flagging blank fields in the registration screen and validity edits for dates and ages.

Medicare and Medicaid Edits

Medicare and Medicaid edits are important parts of any editing program. Similar to the edits that prevent patient access personnel from proceeding with a registration if critical fields are blank, prebilling edits prevent a flawed bill from dropping or from transmitting to the payer. An edit that prevents a bill from dropping occurs before a UB is created. Prebilling edits prevent a bill from dropping before the account is coded. An edit of error identifies problems such as an invalid payer address or national provider identification (NPI) number on the UB and prevents transmission of the UB until the error is corrected. Although all edits could theoretically take place during the prebilling stage, postdrop edits are also used to provide a final look at the account before billing and can catch errors that will delay or prevent reimbursement. For example, HIM staff would not typically see an NCCI edit or MUE on an inpatient record, but patients who have exhausted their Medicare Part A benefits may be alternatively billed under Part B in some circumstances, and additional HCPCS codes or modifiers may be required.

National Correct Coding Initiative Edits

CMS developed the **National Correct Coding Initiative (NCCI)** to promote national correct coding methodologies and control improper coding that leads to inappropriate payment of Medicare Part B claims. The purpose of the NCCI edits is to prevent improper payment when providers report incorrect code combinations. The NCCI contains two tables of edits that include code pairs that should not be reported together for a number of reasons, as explained in the *National Correct Coding Initiative Coding Policy Manual for Medicare Services* (CMS 2016a). Table 7.2 is a portion of an edit table, which has a column for modifiers with three possible scenarios for each code pair. If the number 1 is in the Modifier column, the code pair in columns 1 and 2 is allowed to be billed. However, just because a modifier is allowed does not necessitate its use in every instance. The modifier should only be used in appropriate scenarios. CMS developed its coding policies based on coding conventions defined in the American Medical Association (AMA) CPT manual, national and local policies and edits, coding guidelines developed by national societies, analysis of standard medical and surgical practices, and a review of current coding practices. CMS updates the *Policy Manual* annually (CMS 2016a). Medicare MACs should use the *Policy Manual*

Table 7.2. Column one/column two correct coding edits for CPT Code 17107

Column1 / Column 2 Edits						
Column 1	Column 2	* = In existence prior to 1996	Effective Date	Deletion Date	Modifier	PTP Edit Rationale
				*=no data	0=not allowed	
					1=allowed	
					9=not applicable	
17107	64445		20090401	*	1	Standards of medical / surgical practice
17107	64446		20090401	*	1	Standards of medical / surgical practice
17107	64447		20090401	*	1	Standards of medical / surgical practice
17107	64448		20090401	*	1	Standards of medical / surgical practice
17107	64449		20090401	*	1	Standards of medical / surgical practice
17107	64450		20021001	*	1	Misuse of column two code with column one code
17107	64461		20160101	*	1	Misuse of column two code with column one code
17107	64463		20160101	*	1	Misuse of column two code with column one code
17107	64470		20021001	20091231	1	Misuse of column two code with column one code
17107	64475		20021001	20091231	1	Misuse of column two code with column one code
17107	64479		20090401	*	1	Standards of medical / surgical practice
17107	64483		20090401	*	1	Standards of medical / surgical practice
17107	64486		20150101	*	1	Misuse of column two code with column one code
17107	64487		20150101	*	1	Misuse of column two code with column one code
17107	64488		20150101	*	1	Misuse of column two code with column one code
17107	64489		20150101	*	1	Misuse of column two code with column one code
17107	64490		20100101	*	1	Misuse of column two code with column one code
17107	64493		20100101	*	1	Misuse of column two code with column one code

Table 7.2. Column one/column two correct coding edits for CPT Code 17107 (Continued)

17107	64505		20090401	*	1	Standards of medical / surgical practice
17107	64508		20090401	*	1	Standards of medical / surgical practice
17107	64510		20090401	*	1	Standards of medical / surgical practice
17107	64517		20090401	*	1	Standards of medical / surgical practice
17107	64520		20090401	*	1	Standards of medical / surgical practice

Source: CMS 2016c. CPT codes © American Medical Association 2015. All rights reserved.

Column 1 / Column 2 edits: A code from Column 1 may not be allowed in the presence of the corresponding code from Column 2. If a modifier is allowed to correct the issue, a 1 will appear in the Modifier column. If the codes are determined to be correct, the modifier must be used to make the correction.

as a general reference tool that explains the rationale for NCCI procedure-to-procedure (PTP) edits. Carriers implemented NCCI edits within their claim processing systems for dates of service on or after January 1, 1996.

A subset of NCCI edits is incorporated into the outpatient code editor (OCE) for Hospital Outpatient Prospective Payment System (OPPS) and therapy providers—skilled nursing facilities (SNFs), comprehensive outpatient rehabilitation facilities (CORFs), outpatient physical therapy and speech-language pathology providers (OPTs), and home health agencies (HHAs) billing under types of bills (TOBs) 22X, 23X, 75X, 74X, and 34X.

Medically Unlikely Edits

CMS developed medically unlikely edits (MUEs) to reduce the paid-claims error rate for Medicare Part B claims. An MUE for a CPT/HCPCS code is the maximum units of service that a provider would report under most circumstances for a single beneficiary on a single date of service. Not all CPT/HCPCS codes have an MUE. Table 7.3 includes examples of codes and the maximum number of units Medicare allows based on the need to implement MUEs. MUEs were implemented January 1, 2007, and are used to adjudicate claims at carriers, FIs, and durable medical equipment (DME) MACs (CMS 2016b).

Resources for Editing and Correcting Claims

Providers can find information on CMS-related edits on the CMS website. Please see Resources at the end of this chapter for links to CMS edit tables for National Correct Code Initiative (NCCI), medically unlikely edit (MUE), Outpatient Code Editor (OCE) and Medicare Code Editor (MCE) rules. Payer-specific edit tables can be found on each payer's website.

Many other resources are available to individuals who are responsible for correcting claims. Medicare publishes its claims processing and other manuals online. The MACs also maintain websites with claims tools. In addition, there are a number of vendors who have integrated claims documentation into their codebooks and encoders. Although other payers may have their own mandates for compliance, NCCI edits are Medicare-specific.

Working Failed Edits

When a claim fails on edit, the clock starts ticking to file a timely claim. Timely filing requirements vary by payer and can easily range from 30 days to 180 days. Individuals who work on these

Table 7.3. Selected medically unlikely edits (MUEs)

CPT/HCPCS Code	Hospital Outpatient Service MUE
0016T	2
0017T	2
0019T	1
0030T	2
0054T	2
0055T	2
0064T	1
0067T	1
0071T	1
0072T	1
0073T	2
0084T	1
0085T	1
0087T	1
0099T	2
0100T	2

Source: CMS 2016b. CPT codes © American Medical Association 2015. All rights reserved.

edits are typically PFS personnel. However, since coding can be a major edit issue, HIM personnel are often involved as well.

Even when claims are not coded in the HIM department, working on these edits is an excellent task for an HIM professional housed either in the HIM department or PFS. Correction of these errors is a multipart process. A key component in the correction process is to communicate the error to the department that made it. If errors are merely corrected, it is highly likely that the error will be repeated. Table 7.4 illustrates the process.

Reimbursement and Contract Management

As discussed in chapter 3, contracts with individual payers will likely specify different reimbursement amounts. Some contracts will contain very specific language regarding diagnosis-related groups (DRGs), diagnoses, or procedures. Some payers mirror Medicare UB requirements whereas others use the UB form but have their own requirements regarding the use and importance of each field. For example, a Medicaid payer may require an *International Classification of Diseases, Tenth Revision, Procedure Coding System (ICD-10-PCS)* procedure code on same-day surgical procedures whereas a commercial carrier may not. From an HIM perspective, all records can be coded to the highest degree of specificity as coders are not hampered by payer considerations. It is important to recognize that "Outpatient cases are not typically coded with ICD-10-PCS codes. However, some payers may require them. Those payers should be known to the coders, and the organization needs to have a policy for this type of situation. The question for the organization becomes, do all outpatient cases receive CPT/HCPCS *and* ICD-10-PCS codes, or are ICD-10-PCS codes only applied to those payers requiring them?" (Handlon 2015).

Table 7.4.   Correcting a billing error when a diagnosis of iron-deficiency anemia (D50.9) does not support outpatient radiology account's claim for hip x-ray

Step to Correct Billing	Documentation or Corrective Action
Review physician order to determine reason for test.	Script states x-ray hip R/O fx.
Review radiology report to validate service.	Radiology report exists; hip was x-rayed.
Communicate with the department that coded the account (typically patient access, radiology, or health information management).	Radiology department registered the patient and erroneously typed "S40.851" rather than "S42.851."
Correct the error in the system.	Radiology corrects code in hospital system.
Correct the claim.	Patient accounting corrects claim.
Release the claim.	Patient accounting releases the claim.
Log error and resolution for tracking purposes if the scrubber does not do that.	Patient accounting enters resolution into tracking system.

Payer Identification

The payer at registration may not be the payer at discharge. For example, a patient may present an expired insurance card at registration and provide current information at a later date. A patient may list a commercial payer at registration but later provide identify Medicare as a primary or secondary payer. A patient with no identification may be listed as self-pay at registration but later qualify for Medicaid or a government-funded charity care program. Whether charity care is run at the state level or at the county level varies by state, but ultimately it is a part of the state Medicaid budget.

The claim scrubber applies edits specific to the claim itself. It applies outpatient edits to outpatient claims and Medicare edits to Medicare claims. Therefore, the identification of the appropriate payer is very important not just for sending the original claim, but also for subsequent billing to secondary payers. A claim may go through smoothly to the primary payer, but fail for the secondary payer.

Expected Reimbursement

It is not unusual for a payer to underpay or overpay a claim. Bearing in mind that payers face the same technological and staffing challenges that providers face, mistakes do occur. Payers do not always update accounts in a timely manner, and errors in data entry or contract interpretation are sometimes made.

In an underpayment situation, the provider is likely to follow-up with the payer to obtain correct payment. Underpayment trends from a particular payer may indicate weaknesses in the payer's system. When seeking corrections, it is therefore efficient to batch claims by error type and discuss an entire batch at once.

When faced with an overpayment, the provider has other considerations. The payer contract may have a look-back clause indicating that the provider is entitled to keep the money if the error is discovered too late. It is common to retain overpayments until the payer demands recoupment (return of the overpaid funds), but this is not good business practice for a number of reasons—not the least of which is that retention of overpayments obscures the true financial performance of the provider. As part of the financial month-end closing process, hospitals review historical data to determine how much money to reserve for potential reimbursement to payers for overpayments.

From a financial accounting standpoint, overpayments are unearned revenue. If they are booked as unearned revenue (a liability), then at least there is a record of the overpayment that offsets the incorrect increase in cash and net income will be correct. If overpayments are booked purely as a reduction of A/R, then that asset is understated and net income is overstated. This error is compounded as decisions are made based on the erroneous data. The payer may audit the records, find the error, and demand repayment the next year, which will cause periodic net income to be understated in the repayment period. Therefore, it is important for providers to have policies and procedures to reconcile payments with expected reimbursement, properly account for incorrect payments, and follow-up diligently to resolve erroneous payments. Such policies and procedures should define exactly how each type of erroneous payment will be handled and in what time frame.

Credit Balances

Credit balances are a key performance indicator (KPI) that must be monitored as part of revenue cycle best practice principles. A credit balance is what the hospital has determined to be money owed to a payer. Credit balance reports need to be reviewed daily because both Medicaid and Medicare have very short and specific time frames for paying back an overpayment. Providers cannot wait for Medicare or Medicaid to request a credit balance refund. Medicare requires that the designated signer (per the Medicare application process, generally the chief financial officer or chief executive officer) must affirm quarterly that no outstanding credit balances are owed to Medicare. Generally, credit balances are paid back to Medicare and Medicaid via their electronic access system.

Per the 2012 Affordable Care Act (ACA), providers are to treat managed Medicare and managed Medicaid credit balances the same way they treat Medicare and Medicaid credit balances. The conflict for managed Medicare and managed Medicaid can begin when the provider determines that this type of payer owes the provider for underpayments. A settlement must be documented to show that the contract language has been reviewed and federal regulations have been followed. Generally, with these types of payers, to ensure compliance to both the contract as well as federal and state regulations, it is best to proceed claim by claim to resolve any open over- or underpayment issues instead of seeking a claims settlement.

Other commercial payers follow the payment and audit provisions in their individual contracts with the hospital. A state's health maintenance organization (HMO) or other managed care regulations may include a regulation that addresses overpayments (credit balances) for fully insured accounts. By default, the state language ends up being used for that payer's self-insured accounts, too, which makes implementation and auditing easier for the hospital and for the payer. The managed care team should maintain a grid that tracks each payer's audit-clause time period and how the payer can recoup overpayments. Most states have a look-back period of 12 to 24 months. If the payer and provider have not contractually agreed on a look-back period and state regulation does not prevail, then the look-back period would be based on basic contract law requirements, which could be up to seven years depending on the state regulations for the facility. A provider should look to its own state for basic contract law provisions.

Depending on state regulation and what was agreed to in the audit-and-payment clause of the contract between the payer and provider, the payer may be allowed to recoup money by withholding the amount due against future payments. Generally, state regulations require that the payer send a notice giving the provider 30 to 45 days to respond regarding the money owed to the payer and stating whether the recoupment can be made against future payments. If the provider and payer do not agree money is owed or that recoupment against future payments can be made, then the payer must send a written response per the notice requirements in the general contract provisions.

The revenue cycle team needs to set an acceptable dollar range for daily credit balances. A permissible age of credit balances should also be determined. These figures can vary greatly among providers, depending on the size and financial health of a hospital or health system.

Denial Management

Despite all efforts by the provider to send a clean claim, payers deny claims on many occasions (see figure 7.2). As has been noted, claims may be denied because the patient is not covered for the service provided or the service was not deemed medically necessary. For elective surgeries and procedures or other visits requiring precertification, providers should be aware of the risk of denials and can require a deposit from the patient. In other cases, such as emergency services, the potential for denials may not be known.

Other reasons for denials include technical issues, such as duplicate claims or claims whose dates of service overlap other claims. Most denials related to technicalities are entirely preventable. For example, codes used for diagnoses seen in women only should not be found in records for male patients. Occasionally, the code is correct, but the patient was incorrectly registered. Providers should strive to have a denial rate of 5 percent or lower. In the authors' experience, best practice is a denial rate of 2 percent or lower, which is achievable if all necessary pieces of the revenue cycle process are in place.

Not all denials are necessarily bad. A secondary payer is commonly used to cover services not included in the primary payer's benefit package. In this case, the denial from the primary payer would allow the provider to bill the secondary payer. However, depending on the primary payer's denial reason and the secondary payer's policies, the secondary payer may also deny payment (for example, if the primary payer denied the claim for lacking authorization and the secondary also requires authorization). As noted in chapter 4, for each claim, it is extremely important to verify a patient's benefits from all of his or her payers.

Root Causes of Bill Holds and Denials

If a provider has the resources and willingness to perform extensive cleanup of processing, charging, and coding errors to achieve a clean claim after the discharge and bill-hold period, that provider may not prioritize investigation of why claims are in error. However, for most providers, the back-end claim scrubbing activity is unnecessarily expensive. Therefore, performance improvement plans should be implemented to identify and correct processing flaws that create bill errors. Virtually any performance improvement methodology can be used; however, lean methodologies

Figure 7.2.   Common reasons for denial of reimbursement

- Beneficiary not covered (technical/administrative denial)
- Coordination of Benefits (COB) (technical/administrative denial)
- Medical necessity (medical necessity denial)
- Not reasonable and necessary (medical necessity denial)
- Service provided not covered (technical/administrative denial)
- Duplicate billing (technical/administrative denial)
- Unbundled code (technical/administrative denial)
- Modifier not provided (technical/administrative denial)
- Timely filing (technical/administrative denial)
- Diagnosis procedure code doesn't match service provided (technical/administrative denial)
- Procedure code doesn't match patient sex (technical/administrative denial)
- Procedure code inconsistent with the modifier used (technical/administrative denial)
- Procedure code inconsistent with place of service (technical/administrative denial)
- Diagnosis is inconsistent with age, sex, procedure, etc. (technical/administrative denial)

Source: HFMA 2002. Reprinted with permission. http://www.hfma.org/.

should be taken into consideration. In terms of internal control, it makes sense to develop and implement preventive controls only if they are more efficient and effective than detective and corrective controls. For example, it would usually be more expensive to employ three individuals to screen all charges for data-entry errors than to employ one individual to detect and correct errors at the end of the billing process. Each provider must evaluate the processes that are in place and the limitations of the individuals and systems employed to determine what strategy is best in a given situation. A provider may make different decisions in different departments, depending on the available resources.

Performance Improvement Activity

A review of the claims-error history is the first step in analyzing whether there is a correctable issue. The error history should be sorted by type of error, source of error, timing of error, and specific edit, if applicable. Tables 7.5 and 7.6 present data in a claims-error review.

For each type of error, account-level detail, such as that presented in table 7.6, should be reviewed to determine whether there is a pattern of errors, such as for a specific clinical service, unit, registrar, or coder. Even isolated, seemingly random errors should be followed-up. For example, a single registrar error of an invalid diagnosis code may lead to the discovery that the look-up table in the registration system contains an error. Failure to investigate would allow this error to happen repeatedly.

In the first case shown in table 7.6, assume that the charge clerk had accidentally used an old "cheat sheet" in charging for the echocardiography services. In the other three cases, assume that a new dialysis nurse had entered charges for transfusion administrations that took place during dialysis. Without follow-up, these errors would continue to occur. A few minutes of investigation and re-education would prevent the errors going forward.

Table 7.5. Reviewing claims errors

Error	Description	Number of Claims	Total Charges
Medical necessity	The CPT/HCPCS codes for services on the claim are not supported by the ICD-10-CM diagnosis code.	15	$165,439
Missing modifier	A combination of two or more CPT/HCPCS codes on the claim requires additional information in the form of a modifier.	14	$ 23,678
Invalid diagnosis code	The ICD-10-CM diagnosis code used is not found on the list of codes valid for the dates of service.	8	$ 15,839
Unbundling	A CPT/HCPCS code is used in conjunction with a second CPT/HCPCS comprehensive code that includes the first code.	4	$ 11,804

Table 7.6. Detail of the four unbundling coding errors from table 7.5

Account	Admission	Discharge	Charges	Service	Resolution
6548723456	8/05/09	8/05/09	$ 1,523	Cardiology	Follow-up education provided
6548723367	8/03/09	8/03/09	$ 3,427	Dialysis	Follow-up education provided
6548723423	8/05/09	8/05/09	$ 3,427	Dialysis	Follow-up education provided
6548723567	8/06/09	8/06/09	$ 3,427	Dialysis	Follow-up education provided
Total charges			$11,804		

The best tools for processing claims are those that streamline the revenue cycle and provide feedback to the clinical and administrative players. Key components of useful tools include the following:

- Education of front-end users as well as back-end analysis personnel
- Preventive front-end validity and audit controls
- Tracking of denials, both to ensure timely appeals and to analyze errors for performance improvement
- Feedback to front-end users for correction and performance improvement
- Reporting mechanisms to support organizational and objectives

One way to benchmark for improvement is to review the Comprehensive Error Rate Testing (CERT) reports available on the CMS website. Table 7.7 is an example of a CERT report.

Check Your Understanding 7.2.

1. Distinguish between NCCI edits and MUEs.

2. What are some common reasons for additional handling of claims postbilling?

3. Why are overpayments a problem for providers?

Audits and Denials

Not all denials come immediately after billing. A payer may not analyze payment data for years and then go back to audit and potentially recoup reimbursements. As mentioned in chapter 3, hospitals should pay special attention to certain contract clauses and ensure that impacted departments are aware of the agreed-upon contractual parameters. Audit and denial provisions are no exception. The PFS team needs to know each payer's contractual arrangement as well as the payers' policies as they relate to audits and denials. Most states have managed care regulations that allow for a 12- to 24-month look-back period on credit balances. Generally, contracts specify that these look-back periods apply to all accounts (self-pay as well as fully insured) in the contract for ease of collaborative relationships between the payer and the provider. If the hospital is in a state that does not have managed care regulations, then payers and providers need to negotiate look-backs for denials and credit balances as part of their contract. Look-backs vary widely among payers and programs. The federal **recovery audit contractor (RAC)** program—a governmental program whose goal is to identify improper payments (overpayments or underpayments) made on claims of healthcare services provided to Medicare beneficiaries—has a look-back period of three years.

Providers must have policies and procedures in place to specify how denials will be handled because audit clauses in the contract language for managed care payers are very different than the policies that govern denials. Part of the policy should be specific time frames in which appeals will be handled, as well as dollar thresholds below which an appeal is not pursued. The authors strongly advise that providers use an outside vendor to help ensure that denials are reviewed and pursued in a timely manner. Unless a facility has a dedicated staff person in a managed care or case management department who only works on denials, the organization will not have sufficient time to correctly file and follow up on appeals. In the authors' experience, many providers see a minimum success rate of 65 percent for appeals when the work is outsourced to a vendor or consultant. The same or higher rate of success is difficult for internal staff to achieve.

Outpatient denials are generally technical or administrative denials, although medical necessity denials can occur on an outpatient basis. In contrast, most inpatient denials are for medical necessity. All payers have formal policies and procedures, including time frames, for

Table 7.7.   Paid claims error rate by error type

Type of error	1996	1997	1998	1999	2000	2001	2002	2003	2004	2005	2006	2007	May 2008
	Net	Net	Net	Net	Net	Net	Net	Net	Gross	Gross	Gross	Gross	Gross
No documentation errors	1.9%	2.1%	0.4%	0.6%	1.2%	0.8%	0.5%	5.4%	3.1%	0.7%	0.6%	0.6%	0.3%
Insufficient documentation errors	4.5%	2.9%	0.8%	2.6%	1.3%	1.9%	1.3%	2.5%	4.1%	1.1%	0.6%	0.4%	0.5%
Medically unnecessary errors	5.1%	4.2%	3.9%	2.6%	2.9%	2.7%	3.6%	1.1%	1.6%	1.6%	1.4%	1.3%	1.3%
Incorrect coding errors	1.2%	1.7%	1.3%	1.3%	1.0%	1.1%	0.9%	0.7%	1.2%	1.5%	1.6%	1.5%	1.4%
Other errors	1.1%	0.5%	0.7%	0.9%	0.4%	−0.2%	0.0%	0.1%	0.2%	0.2%	0.2%	0.2%	0.2%
Improper payments	13.8%	11.4%	7.1%	8.0%	6.8%	6.3%	6.3%	9.8%	10.1%	5.2%	4.4%	3.9%	3.7%
Correct payments	86.2%	88.6%	92.9%	92.0%	93.2%	93.7%	93.7%	90.2%	89.9%	94.8%	95.6%	96.1%	96.3%

Source: CMS 2015b.

processing appeals. If a hospital is not a participating provider with a given payer, then the provider can consider suing or filing arbitration to look for a remedy outside the scope of the payer's formal appeals processes. State regulations of managed care also often allow for a state level appeal, which generally includes a fee to file and a state arbitration process. The state appeal processes are intended only for fully insured accounts.

Appealing Medicare Denials

The time frames for appeals are clearly defined for Medicare claims. Copies of documentation to support the appeal are generally necessary. Table 7.8 summarizes the Medicare fee-for-service appeals process. Levels of appeals are available as long as the appeal is filed promptly. Details of the appeal process are available on the CMS website (CMS 2015b). An organization's policies and procedures for denials management should clearly specify exactly how to determine whether an appeal should be made. Some providers, such as large hospitals with high volumes of accounts, may set a dollar limit, such as $50, for denials that are not to be pursued. Other providers, such as physicians, may choose to pursue every possible denial. Some denials, such as for duplicate charges, are not eligible for appeal. However, denials for medical necessity may be successful with some analysis, documentation, and effort.

Tracking and Trending Denials

As any provider with a successful appeals process can attest, persevering through each level of a payer's appeals processes will yield the best overturn rate and allow the provider to gather information about improving internal processes so that denials do not occur in the first place. The provider should be aware of any state regulations that allow a provider to appeal to a state-selected

Table 7.8. Medicare fee-for-service appeals process

Appeal Level	Time Limit for Filing Request	Monetary Threshold to Be Met
1. Redetermination reviewed by the Medicare Administrative Contractor (MAC)	120 days from date of receipt of the initial determination notice	None
2. Reconsideration reviewed by the Quality Improvement Council (QIC)	180 days from date of receipt of the redetermination	None
3. Administrative law judge (ALJ) hearing	60 days from the date of receipt of the reconsideration or after the applicable QIC reconsideration time frame to respond has not been met.	Yes*
4. Departmental Appeals Board (DAB) review/Medicare Appeals Council review	60 days from the date of receipt of the ALJ hearing decision or after the expiration of the ALJ time frame to respond has not been met.	None
5. Federal court review done by the U.S. District Court	60 days from date of receipt of the Appeals Council decision or declination of review by DAB or after the expiration of the Appeals Council time frame to respond has not been met.	Yes*

*Beginning in 2005, for requests made for an ALJ hearing or judicial review, the dollar amount in controversy requirement increased by the percentage increase in the medical care component of the consumer price index for all urban consumers (US city average) from July 2003 to the July preceding the year involved. Any amount that is not a multiple of $10 will be rounded to the nearest multiple of $10.

Source: CMS 2014.

third party to review the appeal if a payer's internal processes have been exhausted. With the permanent implementation of the Medicare RAC program, the importance of a strong denials management program has been highlighted. Organizations may handle their denials internally. If so, the RAC program increases the staff's workload. If the organization outsources denials management, it may choose to outsource this aspect of RAC support as well. Either way, HFMA has some tips for denial management, which are listed in figure 7.3.

To measure the success of the denials management program, the number of claims appealed should be compared to the total denials, and the number of successful appeals should be compared to the number of claims appealed. Denials and appeals should be examined by payer and trends over time should be analyzed. If specific payers are problematic or unreasonable, executive management should intervene. There is little advantage to having a contract with a managed care organization if there are excessive, unreasonable denials. As mentioned in chapter 3, remedies outside of the formal denial appeals process should be included in the contract.

Collections Management

Even if registration, charging, documentation, coding, claim submission and denial management elements are in place and working smoothly, the facility still has to collect the cash it is owed to complete the revenue cycle. In this section, we will discuss the process of analyzing collections and following up on expected cash.

Receipts

Electronic deposits are the simplest way to get cash from the payer into the provider's bank account. Payers do not just send payment; they also send a payment explanation—called a **remittance advice (RA)**, remittance, or remittance notice—that details what claims have been paid. As mentioned earlier in this chapter, these remittances are sent electronically in an 835i (institutional) or

Figure 7.3.   Key components of a denial management program

- Spreadsheet to track status of denials and provide feedback to appropriate person
- Trend denials by CPT/HCPCS code and revenue center
- Involve the attending MD and ask for his/her input prior to submitting [the appeal]
- Keep exact duplicate of everything you send
- Implement tracking by using overnight services or certified mail
- Review and summarize patient history, treatment, progress and P/C [discharge] status
- Address specific denial reasons through process improvement or education
- Cite how patient met regulatory and/or reimbursement guidelines to payer
- Reference attachments to payer
  - Intermediary and carrier guidelines
  - Standards of care
  - Copy of chart
- Track results of claims recovery
  - Denial rate per quarter
  - Turnover rate
- Report claims recovery results with prospective prevention results to PI and corporate compliance officer

Source: HFMA 2002.

835p (physician) format. Historically, these remittances were paper; however, the transition to electronic claim and remittance advice transmission made paper filings unusual. It is up to the provider to reconcile the amount received with the expected payment, as described in the EOB or EOP.

Reconciliation

Let's review an example of reconciliation. In this case, the patient charges total $10,000. The payer contract states that the payer will reimburse 60 percent of charges. The provider submits its claim, and payment of $5,500 is received and posted to the patient's account. Reflecting back to chapter 2, in which we showed the posting of charges, the patient account would look something like this:

Accounts receivable (A/R)	$10,000
Contractual adjustments (CA)	($ 4,000)
Payment	($ 5,500)
Balance	$ 500

Patient accounting must reconcile the $500 balance and determine whether the payment is correct or incorrect. Patient accounting is generally supported in this task by a contract- or reimbursement-management system that automatically reduces accounts to the expected reimbursement upon being billed out during the nightly systems run. As previously discussed in this chapter, the rates are built into the contract- or reimbursement-management system based on the contracted rates as well as the current Medicare and Medicaid rates.

If the payment is incorrect, the payer must be contacted to remit the difference. The difference may be in the interpretation of the contract, which is an issue best resolved early in the relationship between payer and provider. For example, payment for high-cost pharmaceuticals may be reimbursed in addition to the per diem for an inpatient account. If there is an underpayment of the claim, it is possible that the payer neglect to include this portion of the reimbursement. Other possible reasons for the apparent underpayment include the patient's obligation toward a deductible or co-pay, or part of the service may not have been covered. Thus, the analysis and follow-up of receipts is extremely important to ensure that the provider is correctly reimbursed from all possible sources.

Self-Pay Issues

When third-party payer reimbursement is exhausted or there is no third-party payer, the organization may turn to the patient for payment. For Medicare patients, providers can seek self-payment only if the patient has signed an advance beneficiary notice (ABN) for that specific service. For managed care contracts, payers and providers must negotiate self-payment terms in the contract or agree to that such terms will be omitted. Several states have hold-harmless provisions for the fully insured patient population that require the provider to hold the patient harmless (not financially responsible) if the provider renders services that should have been, for example, authorized. Certain scenarios—such as situations when the patient knows an authorization is needed but does not want to wait until it has been obtained or the payer denies authorization because the procedure is not medically necessary—must be discussed and finalized during the contract negotiations. Patients should be able to sign self-pay waivers if they want to receive services in these situations. Similar to the ABN, the self-pay waiver explains that the patient is waiving use of insurance for this encounter.

Patients initially seem to fall in the self-pay category but actually have coverage from private insurance, Medicaid, or Medicare. As discussed in chapter 4, the patient access department is responsible for identifying the patient's means of payment for services. If the patient does not have a relationship with a third-party payer, the patient may be eligible for some government subsidy, often called charity care. Fortunately for providers, since the inception of the ACA, most states have opted to expand their Medicaid programs, allowing more patients to qualify for Medicaid coverage, which helps reduce hospitals' charity care expenses. Furthermore, under ACA, more patients are covered by insurance purchased, sometimes with the help of federal subsidies, on the government's health exchange. It is in the provider's best interests to identify the patient's means of payment before submitting the claim for services. Since the third-party payer will drive the need for a co-pay or other out-of-pocket expenses, which should be collected at the time of service, identification of the payer at registration is best.

Some patients will begin by self-paying for all services. If a patient's self-pay status is known at registration, the facility may request a deposit or offer a discount for self-pay at the time of service. Based on current state or CMS regulations, hospitals may not be permitted to give patients a discount that lowers self-pay rates to less than a certain percentage of current published Medicare rates for their facility. This rule has been further addressed by the Internal Revenue Code (IRC) 501(r) regulations, effective January 1, 2016, that define how not-for-profit providers must handle their self-pay billing and collection policies based on their charity care policy. If a not-for-profit provider is found to be in violation of these regulations, they may lose their not-for-profit status. It is expected that providers are giving a certain amount of care for free as a tax exempt not-for-profit. Payment in full may be requested in advance for elective procedures. The provider should have some process in place to discount charges for self-pay patients and should be able to offer the patient a reasonable payment plan or credit card payment.

It is important to remember that a hospital is contractually obligated to collect the after-insurance amount (self-pay amount) from a patient whether or not the provider is in network with the payer. The patient (member) has a contractual obligation to the payer to pay for services when the hospital is not a participating provider (that is, out-of-network). If a patient does not adhere to the out-of-pocket and out-of-network financial obligation, the payer could say the patient has committed insurance fraud. Additionally, "a provider who routinely discounts or waives a patient's copayment or deductible (collectively referred to as copayment) obligations, for example, can run afoul of the federal anti-kickback statute, 42 U.S.C. § 1320a-7b, or be accused of false billing by private insurance carriers not receiving the discount" (Cohen 2014). Thus, both patients and providers must be cognizant of their contractual obligations, giving providers even more incentive to ensure up-front transparency.

Another self-pay tool that hospitals provide for patients is a secure patient portal. Patients can use a patient portal to access test results or other sections of their medical record, schedule appointments, and pay bills. Bill payment was one of the original reasons for creating patient portals. Patients can pay their after-insurance co-pay, co-insurance, or deductible amount too. The online payment system saves time and money for the patient accounting team because they do not have to be on the phone to take credit card information. Of course, from a customer service perspective, patient portals do not eliminate the need for a PFS customer service center.

There has been abundant discussion in recent years of pricing transparency (disclosure to the patient of the costs of service in advance) (HFMA 2007). For elective procedures, such as plastic surgery, pricing transparency has been in place for many years. However, providing the cost of an emergency department (ED) visit, for example, is not so simple. Prior to delivering ED services, there is no definitive way of determining total charges. A range of prices could be explained, but that range could be many thousands of dollars, which is not helpful to the patient. Further, patients with an emergent medical condition cannot legally be denied treatment or stabilization due to the inability to pay (CMS 2015c). On a practical level, a patient with chest pain is not calling around looking for the lowest-cost emergency care. However, a patient calling about the price of a blood test or an x-ray should be provided with the correct information. An example of pricing transparency is found in some hospitals and physician practices that have developed outreach services in retail stores, such as CVS Minute Clinics (Minute Clinic 2015). These outreach services, while not designed to treat emergencies, provide a low-cost alternative to hospital-based ED visits for minor issues. Their pricing structures are published, which gives potential patients sufficient information to make an informed financial decision.

Bad Debt

Despite transparent pricing and payment arrangements, patients (and payers) occasionally fail to pay what they owe. In such cases, the provider has two options: write off the balance to bad debt or put the debtor into collections.

A write-off to bad debt applies only to accrual-based accounting. If the provider records receivables (and thus revenue) at the time of final billing, then uncollectible amounts can be recorded to reduce A/R and either revenue or a reserve for uncollectible accounts.

Putting a patient into collections for bad debt is a difficult decision, and the hospital's policy should specify whether patients will be reported to the credit bureaus. Despite the underlying purpose of delivering healthcare and its conceptually altruistic foundation, healthcare is a business. Just as theft in department stores drives up the cost of goods, uncollectible accounts drive up the price of healthcare. Thus, it is usually correct to seek payment for services rendered. Sometimes, a final billing notice with a reference to collections is enough to prompt the patient to contact the provider to make payment. More often, the account is referred to a collections agency, which generally receives a portion of the proceeds.

Occasionally, a hospital will choose to sell its bad debt. The cost of collections may be high or the hospital may want to clean up A/R on the balance sheet. Knowing that the debt buyer will be aggressive in collecting payment may cause the provider to hesitate over the potential public relations backlash. Therefore, care must be taken not to include accounts that are under scrutiny for reasons such as patient bankruptcy or provider legal action (HFMA 2004).

HIM professionals who manage a physician or outpatient practice may be involved in accounting for bad debt or bed debt management. They may also encounter bad debt issues if they are involved in patient access functions. HIM professionals may choose to explore opportunities in financial counseling or patient advocacy, which places them in the position of working with both the patient and the provider to work out payment.

Special Considerations for Specific Practice Settings

In general, elective services can be priced and the payment source determined before care is rendered. As with many of the processes discussed in this text, the accuracy of the front-end work will reduce the problems that arise at the back end.

Inpatient Settings

The issues discussed in this chapter are relevant as written to hospital inpatient services. Hospitals are at risk when the payment source is unknown or uncertain before services are delivered. Further, because some services may extend far beyond what is originally predicted—for example, hospitalized patients may be unexpectedly placed on ventilator support—the hospital is exposed to the risk of loss due to uncompensated care. Inpatient accounts are usually high-dollar accounts, and considerable attention is devoted to their claims.

Outpatient Settings

Hospital outpatient accounts may represent a significantly higher volume than inpatient accounts. Therefore, outpatient accounts left unattended may expose the hospital to the risk of loss due to the untimely filing of claims, high rates of errors and denials on claims, and the high cost of correcting low-dollar claims. Under the Emergency Medical Treatment and Labor Act (EMTALA), treatment or stabilization services must be provided to patients with emergent medical conditions, regardless of their ability to pay (CMS 2015c). Since the opportunity to obtain payment information and to collect co-pays may be lost if the patient leaves the ED before relevant payer data are collected, facilities should carefully review the process and patient flow in the ED to maximize cash receipts and provide accurate data collection.

EMTALA does not extend to non-emergent or inpatient care. The hospital must decide, based on resources, community relations, and strategic planning whether to offer these services to patients without a viable means of paying for those services. In not-for-profit facilities, patient care funds may be available from direct contribution or foundation sources for this purpose.

Physician Practices

Physician office practices often post signs stating *payment due at the time of service*. Offices are set-up so that it is difficult, if not impossible, to leave without making arrangements for payment. Since the charge for a physician office visit is relatively low compared to the cost of hospital services, a credit card payment may not be a problem. If physician office staff obtain insurance and patient identification up front, and the insurance is valid, there is not usually a problem being paid. Difficulties arise when the patient is out of plan or has not satisfied a deductible.

Check Your Understanding 7.3.

1. What is a look-back period and why is it important?

2. What are the Medicare fee-for-service appeals process level?

3. What are the key components of a denials management program?

References

Centers for Medicare and Medicaid Services (CMS). 2016a. NCCI Policy Manual for Medicare Services. National Correct Coding Initiative Edits. https://www.cms.gov/Medicare/Coding/NationalCorrect CodInitEd/Downloads/2016-NCCI-Policy-Manual.zip.

Centers for Medicare and Medicaid Services (CMS). 2016b. Medically Unlikely Edits. https://www.cms.gov /Medicare/Coding/NationalCorrectCodInitEd/MUE.html.

Centers for Medicare and Medicaid Services (CMS). 2016c. PTP Coding Edits. National Correct Coding Initiative Edits. https://www.cms.gov/Medicare/Coding/NationalCorrectCodInitEd/NCCI-Coding-Edits.html.

Centers for Medicare and Medicaid Services (CMS). 2015a. Medicare Administrative Contractors as of April 1, 2015. https://www.cms.gov/Medicare/Medicare-Contracting/Medicare-Administrative-Contractors /Downloads/MACs-by-State-April-2015.pdf.

Centers for Medicare and Medicaid Services (CMS). 2015b. National Medicare FFS Error Rate. https:// www.cms.hhs.gov/apps/er_report/preview_er_report.asp?from=public&which=long&reportID=9& tab=4#405.

Centers for Medicare and Medicaid Services (CMS). 2015c. Emergency Medical Treatment and Labor Act (EMTALA). http://www.cms.hhs.gov/emtala.

Centers for Medicare and Medicaid Services (CMS). 2014. Medicare Claims Processing Manual: Chapter 29: Appeals of Claims Decision. Rev. 2926, 04-11-14. http://www.cms.hhs.gov/manuals/downloads /clm104c29.pdf.

Centers for Medicare and Medicaid Services (CMS). 2002. Change Request 2215: Elimination of Official Level III Healthcare Common Procedure Coding System (HCPCS) Codes/Modifiers and Unapproved Local Codes/Modifiers. Program Memorandum Intermediaries/Carriers, Transmittal AB-02-113. https://www.cms.gov/Regulations-and-Guidance/Guidance/Transmittals/downloads/AB02113.pdf.

Cohen, M.K. 2014. Health care providers may waive patients' copayment obligations, but…. *Ober Kaler, Attorneys at Law Legal Perspectives: Health Law Alert.* http://www.ober.com/publications/2472-health-care -providers-may-waive-patients-copayment-obligations-but.

Handlon, L. 2015. Correspondence with authors.

Healthcare Financial Management Association (HFMA). 2007 (October). Pricing Transparency Project Summary Recommendations From HFMA's National Advisory Councils. http://www.hfma.org/NR/rdonlyres /200C8B8E- 0E36-4558-911F-7A170543EA2A/0/400582NACWhitePaperonPricingTransparency.pdf.

Healthcare Financial Management Association. 2004 (August). Bad Debt Rising: When to Sell Your Accounts Receivable. http://www.healthleadersmedia.com/content/138293.pdf.

Minute Clinic. 2015. www.minuteclinic.com.

Additional Resource

Patient Advocate Foundation. 2012. The Managed Care Answer Guide. http://www.patientadvocate.org /requests/publications/Managed-Care.pdf.

Glossary

837i: An electronic transmittal file is transmitted to a data clearinghouse which holds the data until it is released by the facility. While it is being held by the clearinghouse, the facility has the opportunity to review the data in order to identify and correct any errors.

Abuses: Coding errors that occur without intent to defraud the government (for example, a coding rule was not known or updated or was misused).

Account: A subdivision of assets, liabilities, and equities in an organization's financial management system.

Account number: The number patient access assigns to a patient's encounter. It is also called the financial (FIN) number, visit number, or encounter number.

Accounts payable: Records of the payments owed by an organization to other entities.

Accounts receivable (A/R): Records of the payments owed to the organization by outside entities, such as third-party payers and patients, for goods or services provided.

Activity-based costing (ABC): Does not allocate costs but, rather, serves as an economic model that traces the costs or resources necessary for a product or customer.

Admissions: See *Patient registration.*

Advance beneficiary notice (ABN): A document that alerts the patient that if services to be provided are not covered by Medicare, the provider can seek payment from the patient.

Ambulatory payment classification (APC): Hospital outpatient prospective payment system (OPPS). The classification is a resource-based reimbursement system.

Appeal: A request for reconsideration of a denial of coverage or rejection of claim decision.

Asset: Something that is owned or due to be received.

Backlog: A volume of work that has not been completed in the specified time frame.

Balance sheet: A report that shows the total dollar amounts in accounts, expressed in accounting equation format, at a specific point in time.

Bond covenant: The terms of bond issuance.

Bill hold: The waiting period (up to five days for inpatients an up to seven days for outpatients) that allows the provider to reconcile activities versus charges, make corrections as needed, and apply any additional diagnostic and procedural coding.

Bottom line: See *Net operating revenue*

Business record rule: States that a record is admissible as evidence in court assuming documentation occurs in the normal course of business, is recorded by authorized, qualified individuals concurrently with the care provided, and there is no reason to suspect the veracity of the record as presented.

Capitation: A specified amount of money paid to a health plan or doctor. This is used to cover the cost of a health plan member's healthcare services for a certain length of time.

Carve out: Applicable services that are cut out of the contract and paid at a different rate.

Case-mix groups (CMG): The 97 function-related groups into which inpatient rehabilitation facility discharges are classified on the basis of the patient's level of impairment, age, comorbidities, functional ability, and other factors.

Case-Mix Index (CMI): The average relative weight of all cases treated at a given facility or by a given physician, which reflects the resource intensity or clinical severity of a specific group in relation to the other groups in the classification system; calculated by dividing the sum of the weights of diagnosis-related groups for patients discharged during a given period by the total number of patients discharged.

Cash: A short-term (current) asset account that represents currency and bank account balances.

Centralized model: A registrations setup in which registrars report to the patient access department and generally are located in one space or a limited number of spaces.

Charge Description Master (CDM): See *Chargemaster*

Charge: A price assigned to a unit of medical or health service. The price is assigned based on a variety of factors, including cost, payer contracts, and case mix.

Chargemaster: A financial management form that contains information about the organization's charges for the healthcare services it provides to patients. Also called charge description master (CDM).

Claim: A request for payment for services, benefits, or costs by a hospital, physician, or other provider that is submitted for reimbursement to the healthcare insurance plan either by the insured party or by the provider.

Clean claim: A bill devoid of errors and omissions.

Clinical documentation improvement: The process an organization undertakes that will improve clinical specificity and documentation that will allow coders to assign more concise disease classification codes.

Compliance plan: An organization's voluntary strategy to ensure that it complies with all requirements and regulations.

Controllable costs: Costs that can be influenced by a department director or manager.

Corrective controls: Internal controls designed to fix problems that have been discovered, frequently as a result of detective controls.

Cost: The direct or indirect resources used to produce a product or service, either individually or in aggregate.

Cost allocation: The distribution of costs. There are four models or methods: the direct method, the step-down method, the double-distribution allocation, and the simultaneous-equations method.

Cost driver: The activity that affects or causes costs.

Cost object: A product, process, department, or activity for which the healthcare organization wishes to estimate the cost

Credit balance: The amount in a patient account that is less than zero; for example, when reimbursement exceeds the charges in the account.

Credit line: A loan that permits the provider to borrow on an as-needed basis and repay as cash is available.

Data governance: The overall management of the availability, usability, integrity, and security of the data employed in an organization or enterprise.

Data quality standards: The specific organization-based rules that define what data is to be collected, how it will be recorded and edited, and how it will be retained.

Debt: Incurred when money is borrowed and must eventually be repaid.

Decentralized model: Registrars report to the department for which they are registering and may be located in that department.

Denial: When a bill has been returned unpaid for any of several reasons (for example, sending the bill to the wrong insurance company, patient not having current coverage, inaccurate coding, lack of medical necessity, and so on).

Detective controls: Controls that are put in place to find errors that may have been made during a process; for example, routine coding quality audits and registration audits.

Diagnosis-related group (DRG): A classification system that groups patients according to diagnosis, type of treatment, age, and other relevant criteria.

Direct costs: Costs traceable to a given cost object.

Discharged, no final bill (DNFB): The status of patients whose encounters have ended but for whom a final bill has not been prepared.

Emergency Medical Treatment and Active Labor Act (EMTALA): Legislation that states that emergency department patients must be triaged and deemed stabilized before staff attempt to collect insurance information or payment.

Encoder: Specialty software used to facilitate the assignment of diagnostic and procedural codes according to the rules of the coding system.

Encounter: Direct personal contact between a registered outpatient and a clinician or other health care professional for the diagnosis and treatment of an illness or injury from the beginning of a specific group of services to the end of those services.

Equity: The arithmetic difference between assets and liabilities on a balance sheet. Also, the accounts that make up this section on the balance sheet.

Expense: The use of resources in a specified period of time, measured in monetary terms.

Fee for service (FFS): A method of reimbursement through which providers retrospectively receive payment based on either billed charges for services provided or on annually updated fee schedules.

Fee schedule: A complete listing of fees used by health plans to pay doctors or other providers.

Fixed costs: Costs that do not change in response to changes in volume.

Fraud: That which is done erroneously and purposely to achieve gain from another.

Government payer: Third-party insurance providers, such as Medicare and Medicaid, that are run by a government entity.

Grouper: A computer software program the automatically assigns prospective payment groups on the basis of clinical codes.

Home health resource groups (HHRGs): A classification system for the PPS for Medicate home health patient care reimbursement. The groups are determined b OASIS data.

Hospital-acquired condition (HAC): Conditions identified by CMS as "reasonably preventable" in the hospital setting and for which hospitals will not receive additional payment when not present on admission.

Hybrid model: All registrars report to patient access, but they are located in the departments they serve.

Income statement: A report that summarizes an organization's revenue and expense accounts using totals accumulated during the fiscal year.

Indirect costs: Costs that cannot be traced to a given cost object without resorting to some arbitrary method of assignment.

Information governance: The accountability framework and decision rights to achieve enterprise information management. Encompasses both data governance and information technology governance.

Inpatient: A patient who is provided with room, board, and continuous general nursing services in an area of an acute care facility where patients generally stay at least overnight. Requires a physician order to admit.

Inpatient prospective payment system (IPPS): A per case reimbursement system for acute care hospitals based on Medicare severity diagnosis related groups.

Inpatient psychiatric facility DRGs (IPF PPS DRGs): A per diem prospective payment system that is based on 15 diagnosis-related groups, which because effective on January 1, 2005.

Internal controls: Policies and procedures designed to protect an organization's assets and to reduce the exposure to the risk of loss due to error or malfeasance.

International Classification of Diseases, Tenth Revision, Clinical Modification (ICD-10-CM): The diagnosis coding classification system used in the United States since October 1, 2015.

International Classification of Diseases, Tenth Revision, Procedure Coding System (ICD-10-PCS): The procedure coding classification system used in the United States since October 1, 2015, primarily for inpatient procedures.

Inventory: Goods on hand and available to sell presumably within a year (business cycle).

Late charges: Amounts posted to a patient's account after the bill hold period.

Lean methodologies: A system that targets waste and inefficiencies in a process in order to streamline the process itself.

Level charge: The CPT code and price assigned to the unit of medical or health service provided to a patient during a hospital emergency department encounter and related to the intensity of service.

Liability: An amount owed by an individual or organization to another individual or organization.

Master patient index (MPI): A patient-identifying registry used by the patient access department to identify previous encounters and by the HIM department to find records for processing.

Medical identity theft: The fraudulent presentation of a patient for care using someone else's identity or the use of an individual's identity to present fraudulent claims for reimbursement.

Medical necessity: The concept that procedures are only eligible for reimbursement as a covered benefit when they are performed for a specific diagnosis or specified frequency.

Medicare severity diagnosis-related groups (MS-DRG): The DRG system used by Medicare particularly for the inpatient prospective payment system (IPPS).

Medically Unlikely Edits (MUEs): The maximum units of service (by HCPCS/CPT code) that a provider would report under most circumstances for a single beneficiary on a single date of service.

Mortgage: A loan that is secured by a long-term asset, usually real estate.

MPI cleanup: A practice in which duplicate patient records are identified and merged so that the patient is correctly listed under only one number.

National Correct Coding Initiative (NCCI): Developed by CMS to promote national correct coding methodologies and to control improper coding leading to inappropriate payment in Part B Claims.

National Correct Coding Initiative (NCCI) edits: Rules to prevent improper payment when incorrect code combinations are reported. Contains one table of edits for physicians /practitioners and one table of edits for outpatient hospital services, including code pairs that should not be reported together and the maximum likely volume of specific codes (*see* Medically Unlikely Edits) (CMS 2015).

Net income: The condition when total revenue exceeds total expenses.

Net operating revenue: Operating revenue minus operating expenses.

Net loss: The condition when total expenses exceed total revenue.

Notes payable: A financial obligation (liability) that has specific terms of payment in the form of a contract.

Office of Inspector General (OIG) list of excluded individuals/entities (LEIE): OIG has the authority to exclude individuals and entities from Federally funded health care programs pursuant to sections 1128 and 1156 of the Social Security Act and maintains a list of all currently excluded individuals and entities called the List of Excluded Individuals and Entities (LEIE). Anyone who hires an individual or entity on the LEIE may be subject to civil monetary penalties (CMP) (DHHS 2015).

Office of Inspector General's (OIG's) seven elements: Policies and procedures that healthcare organizations should include in their compliance plan.

Outpatient: A patient who receives ambulatory care services in a hospital-based clinic or department.

Outpatient prospective payment system (OPPS): The Medicare prospective payment system used for hospital-based outpatient services and procedures that is predicated on the assignment of ambulatory payment classifications.

Overhead costs: The costs associated with supporting but not providing patient care services.

Patient access: An individual or department of individuals charged with the responsibility of collecting data that initiates the documentation for the patient encounter; also called patient registration or admissions.

Patient identification number: A unique numerical sequence assigned to the patient at the first encounter and is used to identify the patient through all subsequent encounters; also called health record number, medical record number, history number, and chart number.

Patient registration: An individual or department of individuals charged with the responsibility of collecting data that initiates the documentation for the patient encounter; also called registration and admissions.

Patient service revenue: Amounts earned by a healthcare organization attributable to providing services to patients.

Per diem: A reimbursement system based on a set payment for all of the services provided to a patient on one day rather than on the basis of actual charges.

Physician query process policy: A policy that addresses requests from physicians for additional information as part of the coding and reimbursement process.

Plan-do-check-act (PDCA): A performance improvement methodology that serves to improve outcomes through the analysis and amendment of processes.

Post discharge processing: Activities related to documentation, coding, and billing of a patient's encounter or hospital stay.

Preferred stocks: Shares that have a stated dividend rate.

Present on Admission (POA): A condition present at the time of inpatient admission.

Preventive controls: Internal controls implemented prior to an activity and designed to stop an error from happening.

Probationary period: A period of time in which the skills of a potential employee's work are assessed before he or she assumes full-time employment.

Prospective payment system (PPS): A type of reimbursement system that is based on preset payment levels rather than actual charges billed after the service has been provided; specifically, one of several Medicare reimbursement systems based on predetermined payment rates or periods and linked to the anticipated intensity of services delivered as well as the beneficiary's condition.

Receivable: See *Accounts receivable*

Recoupment: Return of overpaid funds.

Recovery audit contractor (RAC): A governmental program whose goal is to identify improper payments made on claims of healthcare services provided to Medicare beneficiaries.

Registration: See *Patient registration*

Relative value unit (RVU): A number assigned to a procedure that describes its difficulty and expense relationship to other procedures by assigning weights to such factors as personnel, time, and level of skill.

Relative weight (RW): Assigned weight that reflects the relative resource consumption associated with a payment classification or group; higher payments are associated with higher relative weights.

Remittance advice (RA): An explanation of payments (for example, claims denials) made by third-party payers.

Resource utilization groups (RUG-III): A case-mix adjusted classification system based on Minimum Data Set assessments and used by skilled nursing facilities.

Resource-based relative value system (RBRVS): A scale of national uniform relative values for all physicians' services. The relative value of each service must be the sum of relative value units representing the physicians' work, practice expenses net of malpractice insurance expenses, and the cost of professional liability insurance.

Retroactive denials: When the provider contacts the payer prior to providing a service, obtains an authorization code, and then is later denied payment.

Revenue: The recognition of income earned and the use of appropriated capital from the rendering of services during the current period (CMS 2013).

Revenue code: Payment codes for services or items in form locator 42 of the UB-04, usually a three or four digit number. Represents the source of the charge, such as: room & board, laboratory, or pharmacy.

Revenue cycle: The series of activities that connect the services rendered by a healthcare provider with the methods by which the provider receives compensation for those services.

Risk: The extent to which the provider's revenues might not cover its costs.

Secured credit: A loan that is based on the value of an *asset* that is owned by the creditor.

Self-pay: Patients who pay for healthcare services themselves when they are either uninsured or when coverage limits are exceeded or the patient is seeking non-covered services.

Severity adjusted long-term acute care diagnosis-related groups (MS-LTC-DRG): Inpatient classification that categorizes patients who are similar in terms of diagnoses and treatments, age, resources used, and lengths of stay. Under the prospective payments system (PPS), hospitals are paid a set fee for treating patients in a single DRG category, regardless of the actual cost of care for the individual. LTC-DRGs are exactly the same as the DRGs for the inpatient prospective payment system (IPPS).

Six Sigma: Disciplined and data-driven methodology for getting rid of defects in any process.

Standard cost profile (SCP): Identifies, analyzes, and defines the activities, including the costs, of departments within the organization to produce a service unit.

Standard treatment protocols (STPs): A component of ABC that identifies the specific service units necessary to produce a given product (patient).

Statement of retained earnings: A statement expressing the change in retained earnings from the beginning of the balance sheet period to the end.

Step-down allocation method: Distributes the costs of nonrevenue, or indirect, departments to other nonrevenue departments and then finally to revenue, or direct, departments.

Stock: Equity securities are shares in the ownership of the organization.

Third-party payer: An insurance company or entity, other than the patient, with whom the patient has a contractual relationship regarding payment for healthcare services.

Total revenue cycle: Average days in DNFB plus average days in accounts receivable.

Unbilled: Specific report that lists patient encounters that have ended but for whom a final bill has not been prepared.

Uncontrollable costs: Costs over which department managers have little or no effect.

Uniform Hospital Discharge Data Set (UHDDS): A core set of data elements adopted by the US Department of Health, Education, and Welfare in 1974 that are collected by hospitals on all discharges and all discharge abstract systems.

Unsecured credit: A loan that is extended based on the overall financial health of the organization and on its credit rating.

Value added: A key component of the Lean methodology in which the positive contributions to a desired outcome are measured. For an action to be value added, it must require no rework (waste), it must change the current state of the service or product to some degree, and the customer must value the action (financially).

Variable costs: Costs that change as output or volume changes in a constant, proportional manner.

Variance analysis: An assessment of a department's financial transactions to identify differences between the budget amount and the actual amount of a line item.

Visit: A single encounter with a healthcare professional that includes all of the services supplied during the encounter.

Workflow assessment: Identifies inefficiencies in a process or system. Volume, quality, and value are key assessment measures.

Answers to Check Your Understanding Questions

1.1.

1. Patient intake, clinical services, charge capture, case management, coding, billing, and collections

2. The patient's medical record supports the charges on the claim.

3. The bill hold is the period of time, usually in days, that the provider has set so that all charges and documentation can be collected before the bill is dropped.

1.2.

1. At the entry level, there are billing- and insurance-related jobs such as medical biller, billing customer service, and collections clerk. The entry-level competencies for HIM programs at the associate-degree level cover the work-based skills needed for these positions. For example, graduates of an accredited associate-degree HIM program can apply and evaluate the application of diagnosis and procedure codes appropriate to settings across the continuum of care; analyze current regulations and established guidelines in clinical classification systems; and evaluate revenue cycle management processes. This training also supports midlevel functions such as coding, clinical documentation improvement, and revenue cycle auditing.

   At the advanced level, baccalaureate-level training in managing data, implementing processes for revenue cycle management, and reporting and applying principles of healthcare finance for revenue management supports practitioners as managers of coding and revenue cycle and in related consulting roles. Ultimately, HIM practitioners with additional training in leadership and strategic models can move into administrative roles.

   Thus, the broad, work-based training that HIM professionals obtain through accredited training programs includes very specific competencies that address revenue cycle management. Therefore, HIM is a logical career path for practitioners with an interest in the revenue cycle. HIM professionals also collaborate with professionals in PAS, PFS, and the medical staff office to support revenue cycle activities.

2 • Optimizing revenue—Efficient charge capture and correct billing for services
• Timely billing—Coding and billing on a timely basis
• Increasing collections—Making sure that all monies owed to the organization are collected

3 Quality assurance, PDCA, Six Sigma, and Lean methodologies. Also, workflow assessment and ISO standards are relevant to performance improvement.

2.1.

1 See table 2.1. Goods or services are provided, a transaction is recorded, and compensation is remitted.

2 Answers will vary but should address, at a minimum, assets (cash, A/R), liabilities (notes payable), and equity (fund balance).

3 Answers will vary but should address, with an example or two, the equation Assets – Liabilities = Equity. Every transaction has at least two "sides," which increase or decrease the relevant account. For example, receipt of cash in payment of an A/R increases cash and decreases A/R but does not change the overall equation.

2.2.

1 $1.1 million. The beginning balance of $900,000 plus the excess of revenue over expenses of $200,000 equals $1.1 million, which carries over to the unrestricted fund balance.

2 Charges correspond to the services provided to the patient and are accumulated in a patient account. When the patient is discharged, the charges associated with the account are posted to increase A/R and increase patient service revenue. Both A/R and PSR are then adjusted (decreased) by the contractual allowance associated with the payer.

3 A group purchasing contract enables an organization to save money by taking advantage of discounts offered to larger purchasers.

2.3.

1 Numerous factors are involved in providing services, including goods such as medications, personal services such as food, and clinical services such as nursing. Each factor has multiple components and includes the volume and intensity of services provided. Furthermore, general administrative costs, such as computer services, must be factored into calculations.

2 Fixed costs do not change in response to changes in volume. Variable costs change in response to changes in volume.

3 • Step-down allocation distributes overhead costs once, beginning with the area that provides the least amount of nonrevenue-producing services.
• Double distribution allocates overhead costs twice, which takes into consideration that some overhead departments provide services to each other.
• Simultaneous-equations method distributes overhead costs through multiple iterations, allowing maximum distribution of interdepartmental costs among overhead departments.

3.1.

1 The more efficient the revenue cycle process is, the sooner cash is received from the payer. Delays in claims processing delay the availability of cash for operations.

2 For provider, the financial risk of reimbursement is the extent to which the provider's revenues exceed, or do not exceed, its costs. From a payer's perspective, the risk is that the premiums received will not cover the reimbursements for covered services rendered.

3 A prospective payment system is a fee-for-service scheme in which the price for a defined service is predetermined based on a variety of factors related to the healthcare setting. In the inpatient setting, those factors include the diagnoses and procedures associated with the case.

4 Pay for performance provides incentives for meeting specific outcomes criteria, including quality, as well as penalties for failure to achieve benchmarks.

3.2.

1 Fraud is an intentional deceit intended to achieve gain. Abuse is an error that results in gain but was not intentional.

2
1. Written standards of conduct
2. Designation of a chief compliance officer
3. Development and implementation of regular, effective education and training
4. Maintenance of a process to receive complaints
5. Development of a system to respond to allegations of improper/illegal activities
6. Use of audits and other evaluation techniques to monitor compliance and assist in reduction of identified problems
7. Investigation and remediation of identified systemic problems and the development of policies addressing the nonemployment or retention of sanctioned individuals

3.3.

1 Some payers reimburse based on a set percentage of charges in some settings. In other scenarios, charges are largely irrelevant to reimbursement.

2 RVUs represent the resources used to provide a service. Medicare uses RVUs for physician reimbursement.

3 To arrive at a set of terms that enables the provider to obtain reimbursement at the desired level of profit.

4.1.

1 Three of the four key data categories are initiated and many of their elements are completed in patient access.

2 Centralized registration facilitates training, data collection consistency, and compliance, but it may limit flexibility in the registration process. Decentralized registration facilitates flexibility, but it may increase inconsistency in data collection and may affect patient flow.

Hybrid methods of registration take advantage of the best of both centralized and decentralized models, but additional issues may arise in the relationship between patient access and the clinical area.

(3) A name is misspelled; the patient denies prior admission; the patient was previously registered under a different name.

4.2.

(1) Government-issued identification containing a photograph, such as driver's license or passport, is best.

(2) At every visit, at the point of registration.

(3) Front-end transparency refers to the provider educating the patient as to the potential financial impact of planned services prior to the services being rendered.

4.3.

(1) Prior approval requirements are determined in the specific insurance plan. Failure to obtain prior approval may result in denial of payment.

(2) An ABN is a form that explains to a patient, in writing, that a specific service will not be covered by Medicare and how much the patient will be billed if Medicare denies the claim.

(3) Invalid diagnosis codes, missing fields, and invalid dates.

5.1.

(1) Inpatient accounts require a physician order to admit. To a hospital, any patient without an order to admit is an outpatient.

(2) From a revenue cycle perspective, a CDI program helps ensure that clinical documentation is clear for reimbursement support purposes. Ultimately, it improves patient record as a communication tool.

(3) Concurrent analysis of patient records, education of clinical staff, greater collaboration to improve documentation, and more effective tracking of results.

5.2.

(1) A chargemaster or charge description master is a database that contains the product or service details for every product or service offered by the organization for which there is an associated charge. The order-entry system pulls data from the chargemaster to post the actual charges to a patient's account.

(2) As often as needed to keep the data current; at minimum, every time CPT/HCPCS codes are updated.

(3) An exploding charge is a charge in the order-entry system that triggers the posting of multiple lines of charges on the patient's bill. Bundling is the inclusion of multiple services in a single CPT/HCPCS code. If services are bundled, then exploding charges to list the component services would be incorrect and the claim would fail.

5.3.

1. Preventive controls, which deter the error in the first place; detective controls, which find errors after they have been made; and corrective controls, which fix errors and seek to develop controls to prevent them from happening again.

2. Daily reconciliation facilitates early detection of open orders, duplicate orders, and missing orders. All services must be preceded by a physician order, which may be documented electronically or by paper script. Failure to detect and correct errors at this stage will result in missing charges, delayed billing, rebilling, or denials for medical necessity.

3. The discharged no final billed (DNFB), late charges, carve-out reports by revenue code (based on contract rate schedules and CDM build), and payer rules that impact reimbursement (CMS three-day payment window, CMS readmission rule, CMS hospital-acquired conditions rule).

6.1.

1. Access by all parties can be simultaneous in an EHR; whereas only one person at a time can view a paper record.

2. Completion of dictated reports.

3. To obtain documentation in the chart that is needed for coding an accurate and complete record.

6.2.

1. A late charge is any charge posted on a date after which it was supposed to be posted. Timing varies, depending on the type of charges. Late charges can delay billing or cause costly rebilling.

2. Key fields must be accurate to drop a clean claim. Although data in all fields must be correct, some fields are more prone to errors than others and should be scrutinized routinely using computerized tools.

3. Examples: Location-associated charges will not automatically be entered; the wrong charges will be entered.

6.3.

1. Prebilling review, targeted review, and random review for accuracy benchmarks.

2. To establish overall accuracy rates for benchmarking.

3. POA flags secondary diagnoses. Secondary diagnoses that are specified hospital acquired conditions (POA = N) cannot be included in the MS-DRG logic.

6.4.

1. High-risk DRGs; issues identified by OIG audits and CERT reports; errors identified in previous audits.

2. Combining outpatient accounts into inpatient accounts; POA status.

3. Medical necessity and charge capture.

7.1.

1 The MAC handles claims; provides beneficiary and provider service, provider enrollment, reimbursement, and payment safeguards; handles appeals; and performs provider education and training, as well as financial management and information security.

2 Payers will remit the agreed-upon amount, leaving an outstanding receivable balance in the patient's account. Absent any amount due from the patient, the provider will need to adjust the balance to close the account. Without the contractual adjustment, the claim will remain outstanding.

3 Lack of coverage, lack of medical necessity, and billing errors

7.2.

1 NCCI edits prevent improper claims due to inappropriate code combinations. MUEs prevent improper claims due to quantities beyond what would normally billed for an individual in a single encounter.

2 Coding errors, payer identification issues, and incorrect payment.

3 Providers are obligated to return overpayments when they are identified. The time limits on recoupment vary among payers, so the obligation may expire for one payer but not another.

7.3.

1 The look-back period is the contractually agreed-on time during which a payer can recoup reimbursements by denying a provider's claim on retrospective audit. If the provider does not make financial provisions for recoupment, the provider could face disastrous financial consequences.

2 Redetermination; reconsideration; administrative law judge hearing; departmental appeals board (DAB) review/Medicare appeals council review; federal court review.

3 Spreadsheet to track status of denials and provide feedback to appropriate person
- Trend denials by CPT/HCPCS code and revenue center
- Involve the attending MD and ask for his/her input prior to submitting
- Keep exact duplicate of everything you send
- Review and summarize patient history, treatment, progress and P/C status
- Address specific denial reasons through process improvement or education
- Cite how patient met regulatory and/or reimbursement guidelines to payer
- Reference attachments to payer
- Track results of claims recovery

Report claims recovery results with prospective prevention results to PI and corporate compliance officer

Index